Physical Techniques in Cardiological Imaging

Physical Techniques in Cardiological Imaging

Proceedings of the meeting on Physical Techniques in Cardiological Imaging held at the Medical and Biological Sciences Building, University of Southampton, 8–9 July 1982

Edited by M D Short, D A Pay, S Leeman, R M Harrison

Adam Hilger Ltd, Bristol

British Library Cataloguing in Publication Data
Meeting on Physical Techniques in Cardiological Imaging
    (1982: Medical and Biological Sciences Building, University of Southampton)
Physical techniques in cardiological imaging.
1. Cardiovascular systems — Diseases — Diagnosis — Congresses
2. Imaging systems in medicine — Congresses
I. Title   II. Short, M. D.
616.1'7'5   RC670.5.0/

ISBN 0-85274-750-0

The meeting on Physical Techniques in Cardiological Imaging was organised by the Hospital Physicists' Association in liaison with the British Cardiac Society

Organising and Editorial Committee
        M D Short, D A Pay, S Leeman, R M Harrison

Editor in Chief
        M D Short

Published by Adam Hilger Ltd, Techno House, Redcliffe Way, Bristol BS1 6NX, England.

Printed in Great Britain by J W Arrowsmith Ltd, Bristol.

Contents

Preface

In July 1982 a meeting entitled 'Physical Techniques in Cardiological Imaging' was held at the Medical and Biological Sciences Building, University of Southampton. The two-day meeting, organised jointly by the Radionuclide, Physiological Measurement, Diagnostic Radiology and Ultrasound Topic Groups of the Hospital Physicists' Association, was held in liaison with the British Cardiac Society. The aim was to review the physical principles underlying the various imaging disciplines, present clinical overviews and to describe specific state-of-the-art procedures. A discussion of the validity of each type of imaging procedure in specified clinical situations concluded the meeting. The papers contained in these proceedings are the full versions of the presentations at the meeting. In excess of a hundred delegates registered for the meeting which, in addition to the scientific sessions, included a manufacturers' exhibition and scientific poster display. The editors gratefully acknowledge the participation of the following companies.

American Hospital Supply (UK) Ltd
Amersham International plc
Byk-Mallinckrodt (UK) Ltd
CIS (UK) Ltd
Elscint (GB) Ltd
Filtered Air Systems Ltd
International General Electric Company of New York Ltd
Kontron Instruments
Medical Data Systems
Nodecrest Ltd
PMS (Instruments) Ltd
Siemens Ltd
Squibb Medical Systems Ltd
Technicare Imaging Ltd
Toshiba Medical Systems Ltd

A full social programme provided a manufacturers' reception and a conference dinner at historic Beaulieu Abbey which included a visit to the National Motor Museum.

In conclusion, the success of this interdisciplinary cardiological imaging meeting indicated potential for a similar format in the not-too-distant future.

M D Short
D A Pay
S Leeman
R M Harrison
Editors

Imaging in Cardiology: The Cardiologist's Viewpoint

D J Rowlands

University Department of Cardiology, Manchester Royal Infirmary, Manchester M13 9WL

Mr. President, Ladies and Gentleman, when Dr. Short first approached me to open the programme with a general discussion on the viewpoint of the cardiologist on imaging techniques in his own discipline, I anticipated a relatively simple task. I am no longer sure it is so simple. In some ways, of course, it must be easy - all I have to do is to provide a "shopping" list of imaging requirements and then stand well back while the technologists develop and refine the appropriate techniques. When they have finished I can criticise their efforts. On the other hand, if I adopt such an approach I will necessarily be constrained by the limitations of my own experience and imagination. Very often in the past technological advances have suggested to the cardiologist, as to those in other disciplines within medicine, needs which he did not actually realise that he might have. To some extent, therefore, it has to be a two way process. The clinician has to suggest to the technologist some types of information to which he requires access and, at the same time, the technologist has to indicate to the clinician areas of rapid development with increasing access to information which might ultimately prove of clinical value. The hallmark of success must surely be a closely interknit interface rather than a flat boundary zone between the respective disciplines of the clinician and the technologist. Meetings of the type we are now embarking upon offer considerable hope of facilitating the development of just such interfaces. If this conference is a success in this area then it will inevitably follow that any ideas I can put forward at this stage about the cardiologist's view on imaging techniques within cardiology will necessarily be appreciably modified by the time the conference is over. Let us, nevertheless, see what kind of problems face us at this stage.

TABLE I

MAJOR CLINICAL AREAS OF INTEREST TO CARDIOLOGISTS

Coronary Heart Disease
Hypertension
Valvular Disease
Myocardial Disease
Arrhythmias
Conduction Disturbances
Thrombo-embolism
Congenital Heart Disease

Table I represents the major clinical areas of current interest to practising cardiologists. In adult cardiology throughout the western world there is absolutely no doubt that coronary heart disease presents the major challenge both diagnostically and therapeutically. Any advances in acquiring information about this condition will be widely welcomed. The second commonest problem facing the cardiologist today is hypertension. We do not currently tend to think of hypertension as being a fruitful field for imaging but it is always possible that this is one of the inbuilt constraints of which we are ourselves unaware. Who knows, for example, whether future imaging techniques will enable us to see differences in the arterioles or in the myocardium of hypertensive patients. When it comes to valvular disease the pattern is changing appreciably at present. Rheumatic valve disease has been declining very rapidly in developed countries of the world, although there is still a residual pool requiring evaluation and treatment and the continued occurrence of congenital valve disease will ensure that this problem will never completely disappear. Valvular disease has been one important area of application of imaging techniques ever since such techniques have been available and the importance of imaging in the evaluation of valvular disease of the heart is not likely to decline in the future. Primary disease of the myocardium constitutes a relatively rare group of conditions which is nevertheless important because of the often serious prognosis. Much meaningful information about such conditions has already been achieved by imaging processes and further development in this area would certainly be welcome. The arrhythmias and conduction disturbances would not appear to be a potential area for the development of imaging techniques except for the seemingly unlikely possibility that techniques might one day become available which would selectively show the pacemaker and conducting tissue in normality and in disease. Thrombo-embolism lends itself to investigation by imaging methods including isotopic techniques and angiography. Finally, there is the enormously complicated field of congenital heart disease. The days when the same cardiologist looked after patients with acute myocardial infarction and neonates with complex congenital abnormalities are over in developed parts of the world. Very properly the management of congenital heart disease is now localised to just a few centres within the country so the general cardiologist is unlikely to be presented with the need for imaging in congenital heart disease. Nevertheless, the need for highly refined discriminatory tests in this area is particularly acute and great hopes are held out for developments in this field.

TABLE II

MAJOR ROLES OF IMAGING TECHNIQUES

Diagnosis
Screening
Quantification
? Tissue Diagnosis

Table II shows what I consider to be the major roles of imaging in general The most obvious of these is that the technique should provide evidence for the diagnosis of the given condition with greater or lesser degrees of specificity. As with all diagnostic tests the specificity will vary with the prevalence of the condition according to the Baysean analysis. Diagnostic tests need not be non-invasive. However, ideally the techniques should also be useful for screening, that is for demonstrating the diagnosis in the apparently healthy population in the absence of any other signs or symptoms of the abnormality. Screening tests must necessarily be of low invasiveness. In addition, the technique should permit a means of quantifying the extent of the abnormality in any case. Finally it is to be hoped that imaging methods might provide chemical or histological descriptions of tissues to permit the kind of tissue diagnosis currently provided only by biopsy examination.

When a new investigative technique appears in the clinical arena it is usually received from two opposing viewpoints. Those who develop the technique are often inclined to be over-optimistic about its merits. Those not involved in the development may be reluctant to accept its advantages. When a new technique is developed the authors therefore have a responsibility to produce a balanced view of their work. They may do considerable harm by over-enthusiasm in the early stages, particularly since justification of a new procedure always involves comparison with existing techniques. In common, I expect, with many people in the audience, I have been asked on many occasions to referee articles submitted to scientific journals. In this regard, at one stage a whole series of articles appeared comparing the results of exercise stress tests using thallium with those obtained using electrocardiography. I was struck by the disparity between the papers. Some clearly demonstrated the superiority of thallium scanning and some of exercise electrocardiography. The explanation was not hard to find. Those whose work had for some time involved isotopic investigation undertook meticulous studies with thallium and often compared these with single lead exercise electrocardiography. They were inexperienced in the use of the electrocardiogram in exercise and without exception they found the thallium procedure to be better. Conversely, those whose work had for some time involved exercise electro-cardiography undertook meticulous ECG studies using multiple lead systems and compared the results with casual, ad hoc thallium studies. Each group was guilty of bias in the comparison. Such bias is, in the end, futile for the true value and limitations of an investigation usually become apparent with time.

Let us therefore consider the techniques currently in use for imaging in cardiology.

TABLE III

IMAGING TECHNIQUES IN CARDIOLOGY

In Widespread Use

> Plain Radiography
> Contrast Radiography
> Isotopic Technique
> Ultrasound

Under Development

> Computed Tomography
> Digital Radiography
> Nuclear Magnetic Resonance
> Emission Computed Tomography

Table III shows the major investigative techniques. The plain chest X-ray is still the most extensively used imaging technique in cardiology. It has the virtue of being non-invasive, generally available, reproducible and relatively well understood both in its inherent value and for its limitations. In some ways, therefore, it is a standard against which other techniques will be judged. It does, however, have very severe limitations. It tells us the overall cardiac size in 2 dimensions (or, with an additional lateral view, in 3) and a great deal about the pulmonary vasculature but it cannot distinguish between an enlargement due to different cardiac chambers nor cannot, except in the case of an obvious aneurysm, distinguish localised areas of healthy and sick myocardium.

Contrast radiography does, of course, provide selective, highly delineated anatomical information concerning the size, shape and location of the cardiac chambers and major vessels and it also provides physiological information about valvar stenosis and competence and about regional myocardial contractile performance. It is, of course, highly invasive. Contrast radiography is likely to remain the gold standard for other techniques setting out to evaluate overall and regional left ventricular contractile function and the recognition of the extent and distribution of stenosing atheroma in the major coronary vessels. In this respect it has proved itself prognostically. For example, the presence of a 75% or more localised stenosis in the main stem of the left coronary artery is associated with a 60% death rate over 5 years. A similar lesion in the right coronary artery carries a 5-10% death rate.

Isotopic techniques developed relatively late in this country compared with their use in South America and in some European countries but their use is now well advanced. The increased utilization in the U.S.A. and in Europe occurred as a result of the development of the gamma camera with its computer back-up. Static blood pool scanning, ionic tracer scanning, infarct-avid scanning and dynamic blood pool studies are now accepted by cardiologists as established techniques in the investigation of ischaemic heart disease, myocardial disease, valve disease and congenital heart disease. One of the biggest problems of nuclear techniques in general is the relatively poor spatial resolution which currently, at best, seems to involve recognition of tissues no smaller than 0.5 cm   in diameter.

Ultrasound techniques are completely non-invasive and involve no radiation. Furthermore they provide a very high degree of spatial resolution - of the order of 0.5 to 1.0 mm. The drawbacks are the limited windows for access to cardiac study and the difficulty of obtaining good recordings in a significant proportion of patients. The older the patient the less likely it is that an adequate study will be achieved. Real time cross-sectional echocardiography has dramatically enhanced the value of this technique, particularly in the study of congenital heart disease.

There are also several techniques under intensive development. Computed tomography is already well advanced in static imaging of the brain and of the trunk but further development is needed before the full benefits of this technique can be applied to a dynamic structure like the heart. However, it does seem extremely likely that this technique will provide dramatic benefits in cardiac imaging within the next decade. Digital radiography offers the prospect of bringing in the benefits of contrast angiography without the need for highly invasive approaches. Dual-energy

digital radiography can be used to isolate visually a blood vessel
containing low doses of contrast from the surrounding medium and digital-
temporal subtraction can produce spatial resolution which is only slightly
inferior to that currently obtained with conventional high density contrast
injections. Emission computed tomography (using injected or inhaled
radionuclides) suffers from the main inherent problem of all radionuclide
techniques, namely poor spatial resolution, but nevertheless offers the
prospect of providing quantitative information about such things as
regional blood flow, oxygen utilization and extraction and biochemical
activity.

TABLE IV

PLAIN RADIOGRAPHY

Advantages

    Non-invasive
    Extensively used
    Well understood (values and limitations)
    Reproducible

            :- it is a "model" technique

Drawbacks

    Cannot reliably distinguish - various cardiac chambers
                                - sick from healthy myocardium
                                - cardiac cavity, myocardium, pericardial
                                  fluid

TABLE V

CONTRAST RADIOGRAPHY

Advantages

        Selective, high resolution information
        Size, shape and location defined
        Myocardial function assessed
        Valvar stenosis and incompetence demonstrated

                :- it is the "gold" standard

Drawbacks

        Highly invasive
        Involves higher radiation dose

TABLE VI

ISOTOPIC TECHNIQUES

Advantages

    Non-invasive
    Myocardial and valve function assessed
    Myocardial viability demonstrated

Drawbacks

    Limited resolution
    Poor anatomical detail

TABLE VII

ULTRASOUND

Advantages

    Non-invasive
    No significant radiation risk
    High resolution
    Detailed anatomy
    Myocardial function assessed

    :- it is an ideal screening procedure
        for structural defects and is very
        suited to paediatric work

Drawbacks

    Limited zones of access to the heart
    Technically impossible in a proportion
    of patients

The virtues and drawbacks of the four major established techniques are listed in Tables IV to VII.

The clinical cardiologist has, then, already come to rely very heavily on imaging techniques. Some of these are old trusted friends, others are new acquaintances of uncertain long term reliability whose true value will only be shown with the passage of time. New techniques are evolving all the time and refinements of currently available techniques are evolving even more.

TABLE VIII

IMAGING IN CARDIOLOGY: MAJOR REQUIREMENTS

Coronary Heart Disease

    Myocardial pathology - normal, ischaemic, necrotic, fibrotic
    Myocardial function - regional, global, phase relations
    Coronary artery pathology
    Coronary arterial graft pathology

Valvular Heart Disease

    Anatomy
    Function

Congenital Heart Disease

    Anatomy
    Function

The most fruitful areas for cardiac imaging with the current pattern of
disease in Western civilised medicine would appear to be as shown in
Table VIII. Undoubtedly coronary heart disease is going to continue to
present the greatest challenge within the foreseeable future. We are
going to require all the information we can possibly get in the intact
patient on the pathology of the myocardium, needing to distinguish the
normal myocardium, ischaemic myocardium, necrotic and fibrotic myocardium,
on myocardial function both regional and global and also on the phase
relations of functions within different parts of the ventricle, on
coronary artery pathology and on coronary graft pathology. We are going
to continue to need observation about the anatomy and function in cases of
valvular heart disease and we are going to need detailed anatomical and
functional studies in congenital heart disease.

TABLE IX

IMAGING IN CARDIOLOGY: RELEVANT FACTORS

    Invasiveness
    Radiation dose
    Installation costs
    Running costs
    Resolution - spatial, temporal, density
    Information - anatomical, functional,
                     biochemical, pathological

Table IX shows the factors which will inevitably be relevant in the
acceptability or otherwise of imaging techniques as they evolve. The
questions of invasiveness and of radiation are of relative not absolute
importance. There will always be room for the imaging technique which
involves risks to the patient through an invasive approach or through
exposure to radiation but obviously, other things being equal, the less

either of these properties is involved the better. The same applies to the question of cost both in terms of installation and in terms of running costs. We would want the best possible resolution in time and space and also preferably in tissue characteristics such as density and we would want to obtain the greatest amount of anatomical, functional, biochemical and pathological data about each tissue image.

Sometimes we may profit by the use of two or more imaging techniques simultaneously, for example the combined use of plain radiography and cardiac blood pool scanning in the case of congestive cardiomyopathy and the use of plain radiography with ionic tracer scanning in patients with hypertrophic cardiomyopathy.

Ladies and Gentleman, I was asked to present a brief account of the cardiologist's view of cardiac imaging. I suspect that my cardiological colleagues would have preferred the title to refer to a cardiologist and would have regarded the use of the definite article as inappropriate. They should not, however, be too distressed. To be asked to give an overview is a sure and certain sign that one's impending senility has been recognised. I mentioned this fact to my secretary and was distressed to discover that it came as no surprise to her. However, I did point out that one further stage in the degenerative process is possible and that that will have been reached when I finally give a talk entitled, "Whither cardiology?". She is under strict instructions that if I ever agree to give such a presentation she is to have me put down in a kindly fashion.

Perhaps I could usefully conclude by reading you a few lines from "Through the Looking Glass" by Lewis Carroll. They are from the story of the Lion and the Unicorn. The King wished to know if his messengers were visible coming along the road and he said to Alice, "They've both gone to the town. Just look along the road, and tell me if you can see either of them". "I see nobody on the road", said Alice. "I only wish I had such eyes", the King remarked in a fretful tone. "To be able to see nobody! and at that distance too! Why, its as much as I can do to see real people by this light!". Mr. Chairman, Ladies and Gentleman, the cardiologists amongst us await with considerable expectation the development of imaging techniques within the next few years and with considerable interest the deliberations of this conference.

Echocardiography: A Clinical Overview

S Hunter
Department of Cardiology, Freeman Hospital, Newcastle upon Tyne.

1. Introduction

Since Edler (1956) first demonstrated the mitral valve using a primitive
M-mode echo machine, echocardiography has assumed a major role in the
diagnosis of all forms of heart disease. There are few cardiac
abnormalities or lesions which cannot be assessed using ultrasound.
Recently, several authors have argued that many patients may proceed to
surgery without invasive investigations, both those with acquired valvular
heart disease (Sutton et al 1981, Hall et al 1983) and those with
congenital heart disease (Macartney et al 1983). However, catheterisation
and angiography should not, in general, be considered to be in competition
with echocardiography. Haemodynamic data can be achieved <u>directly</u> only
by invasive procedures. Conversely, echocardiography can provide
anatomical and functional data, particularly with regard to inlet valves,
which are not available at invasive investigations.

In this overview, it is possible to describe only briefly the most
outstanding instances where cardiac ultrasound has made a major
contribution.

2. M-mode versus cross-sectional or real-time echocardiography

Many investigators now feel that cross-sectional echo (CSE) has made
M-mode echo (MME) redundant. Nothing could be further from the truth.
Whatever the type of machine (phased array, mechanical sector or linear
array) the advantage of CSE is that a more complete anatomical picture of
the heart is available, relating chambers and great arteries to each other.
Thus, for the identification of ventricular septal defects (Sutherland et
al 1982), or abnormalities of intracardiac connections (Smallhorn et al
1982), the CSE technique is vastly superior. However, the number of
repetitions per second of echo information is much less than for MME,
giving the latter advantages when it comes to providing actual functional
data such as shortening or lengthening rates for the left ventricle
(Gilson and Brown 1973). Accurate measurement of chamber size and wall
thickness is better achieved by MME than by CSE. Timing of cardiac events,
particularly with regard to valvular movement, is much easier
and accurate using MME.

Thus the echocardiographer requires both techniques and most CSE machines
now provide MME using a movable cursor which has an added advantage in
that the siting of the MME cut is accurately known by reference to the
CSE image from which it is derived.

3. Echocardiography in valvular heart disease

The decision to operate on patients with valvular heart disease still
depends on the clinical assessment of the patient. The echo findings
corroborate the presence and severity of the lesions. Some of the
information is available from visual assessment of MME and CSE, but more
sophisticated handling of MME, using digitisation (Gibson and Brown 1973,
Hall et al 1981), can provide very reliable information to support the
clinical diagnosis. Single valve lesions such as mitral stenosis lend
themselves more readily to accurate assessment by echo than do multiple
valve lesions. If the suspicion of coronary artery disease exists then
there are strong indications for invasive procedures (coronary
angiography). Nonetheless, there are now two well documented studies
dealing with the efficacy of non-invasive investigations in valvular heart
disease (Sutton et al 1981, Hall et al 1983). Both studies bear out the
contention that valvular heart disease patients can be safely and
expeditiously handled by non-invasive diagnostic techniques, including
both modes of echocardiography. The benefits to the patient in safety
and comfort, and to the hospital in costs, are very great.

4. Other acquired lesions susceptible to echo diagnosis alone

Several forms of acquired heart disease are already accepted as
diagnosable by echocardiography without any invasive procedure.

Cardiac tumours are quite a common problem in large cardiac centres, the
most common being secondary to lesions elsewhere in the body. In our own
centre, we have recently carried out a study of patients undergoing surgery
for carcinoma of the lung and have been able to demonstrate accurately
pericardial or cardiac cavity involvement in every instance where it
existed. Any competent echocardiographer gains satisfaction from
diagnosing the commonest primary tumour of the heart, the atrial myxoma,
which is commonly left sided although occasionally found on the right.
These tumours were regularly diagnosed by MME and are beautifully
delineated by CSE. No further investigation is necessary before surgery.
Even intra-mural tumours can be recognised (Sutherland et al 1980), the
most common being the rhabdomyoma, Most intra-cavitary cardiac tumours are
recognised because they present dense echoes where none should be.
Similar appearances can be seen with organised intra-cavitary clot,
particularly if pedunculated.

This brings us into the realm of tissue recognition, a long promised but
as yet unrealised dream of echocardiographers. Undoubtedly, CSE can
demonstrate pathological changes in tissues such as fibrosis in myocardial
infarction and calcification on a mitral valve. Recently, the use of
colour allied to grey-scale settings using an encoder has provided clearer
differentiation of fibrosis or infiltration of the myocardium (Logan-
Sinclair et al 1981). Tissue recognition may well be available to
echocardiographers in the future.

Cardiomyopathies are the next group of cardiac diseases which can be
diagnosed and followed up by ultrasound. Whether hypertrophic,
obstructive, dilated or secondary to virus myocarditis, the features are
well described and reliable (Roelandt et al 1982). Asymmetric   septal
hypertrophy, systolic anterior movement of the mitral valve anterior
leaflet and mid-systolic closure of the aortic valve are all usually
found in hypertrophic obstructive cardiomyopathy (HOCM).

Doubt persists in two areas. Assymetric septal hypertrophy exists in
other lesions, coarctation of the aorta, systemic hypertension, aortic
stenosis and right ventricular hypertrophy. Systolic anterior movement
of the anterior mitral leaflet may also be found in systemic
hypertension and any condition with a small abnormally shaped left
ventricular cavity. However, the combination of all the above features
reliably diagnoses HOCM, particularly when set against the background
of clinical, radiological and electrocardiographic findings.

Dilated cardiomyopathy at all ages of life is easily recognised by gross
dilatation of the left ventricle with poor contraction, and a large
systolic dimension. The aetiology of the dysfunction is harder to determine
and it is not possible in many instances to differentiate between end-
stage ischaemic heart disease and dilated cardiomyopathy from the echo
findings alone. All the features described so far are easily attainable
by MME. CSE does help to confirm that the whole of the left ventricle
is dysfunctional (in dilated cardiomyopathy) or that the septum is
specifically hypertrophied in HOCM.

Another acquired cardiac disease which lends itself specifically to
echo diagnosis is pericardial effusion. There is now no valid reason to
resort to any other method for this diagnosis. Reliable visualisation of
pericardial fluid,whatever the case and whatever its amount, is
available from both modes of echo. Usually CSE is more informative than
MME, and allows appreciation of the extent of the effusion as well as
identifying deposits or adhesions within the pericardial space.

5. Congenital heart disease

It is for this aspect of cardiology that CSE has produced the greatest
benefits. Its ability to visualise several chambers and their relationships simultaneously is vital. Undoubtedly in this field, the number of
invasive investigations has been greatly diminished by CSE and
specific anatomical information is available which may be unobtainable
with invasive studies. So vast is this subject that the reader can
only be recommended an appropriate monograph (Silverman and Snider 1982)

The simple lesions are easily visualised. We have studied a large group
of children with ventricular septal defects (Sutherland et al 1982). The
accuracy of the technique permits differentiation of ventricular septal
defects according to their situation in the relative parts of the
ventricular septum, inlet, outlet, trabecular and membranous. Assessment
of the size of ventricular defects using CSE and clinical features can
be very accurate and it appears that recognition of the site of the lesion
can help the clinician to predict the natural history of the defect.
For instance, a trabecular (muscular) ventricular septal defect has a
greater chance of closing than a subaortic or inlet ventricular septal
defect.

Abnormalities of the interatrial septum are well visualised with CSE.
Deficiencies of primum and secundum septa are readily differentiated
on four-chambered subcostal views. The apical four-chambered view,
because it lies parallel rather than at right angles to the interatrial
septum, may show artefactual echo drop-out, wrongly suggesting an atrial
septal defect. The fact that the primum atrial septal defect and the
complete atrioventricular septal defect (AV Communis) are the same basic
lesion is beautifully demonstrated by CSE. Both have a common

atrioventricular valve structure straddling from one lateral AV sulcus to the other. Usually, the primum atrial septal defect has only an atrial defect while the complete form has a ventricular component as well. The latter form frequently has a common orifice in the atrioventricular valve tissue whereas the former almost always has two orifices (Anderson et al 1982).

CSE has revolutionisedthe assessment of ventricular arterial connection abnormalities (Silverman et al 1982). Using a multi-window approach, a combination of parasternal long-axis, apical long-axis and subcostal four-chamber plus aortic root views are employed. The ventricles and the great arteries are reliably identified by CSE and then their connections demonstrated by angling from ventricles to arteries. In biventricular hearts, ventricles are recognised echocardiographically by their inlet valves, bileaflet, paired papillary mitral valve and bileaflet single main papillary tricuspid valve. The great arteries are identified by their branching pattern, early bifurcation in the pulmonary artery and late branching non-bifurcation in the aorta. Thus, transposition of the great arteries, Fallots's tetralogy, double outlet right ventricle and truncus arteriosus are all reliably diagnosed by CSE.

The suprasternal approach was useful in congenital heart disease even when only MME was available (Hunter et al 1982). With the advent of CSE the approach has yielded very vital information about congenital heart disease. Coarctation of the aorta can be observed in infancy in a long-axis plane and, if combined with the short-axis view, the presence of a ductus arteriosus can also be shown. In our experience, we can frequently dispense with aortography in infants with coarctation syndrome, thus obviating a source of morbidity in this rather sick group.

6. Summary

In this short paper it has only been possible to describe briefly the clinical usefulness of echocardiography; the literature is now voluminous. Although both MME and CSE are still of great value, the echocardiographer must evaluate the echo findings in association with clinical, radiological and electrocardiographic findings. This point can not be stressed too strongly, for to practice echocardiography 'in a vacuum' is to court disaster!

References

Anderson R H, Ho S Y, Becker A E and Tunan M 1982
The echocardiographic anatomy of congenital heart disease
Echocardiography One, Ed Hunter S and Hall R J C
(Churchill Linvingstone: Edinburgh)

Edler I 1956
Ultrasound Cariogram in mitral valve disease
Acta. Chir. Scand 111 230

Gibson D G and Brown D J 1973
Measurement of instantaneous left ventricular dimension and filling
rate in man using echocardiography
Br. Heart J. 35 1141

Hall R, Austin A and Hunter S 1981
M-mode echogram as a means of distinguishing mild and severe mitral
stenosis
Br. Heart J. 46 486

Hall R J C, Kadushi O A and Evemy K 1983
Is cardiac catheterisation necessary in the assessment of patients
for valve surgery?
Echocardiography Two, Ed by Hunter S and Hall R J C
(Churchill Livingstone: Edinburgh) to be published

Hunter S, Sutherland G and Mortera C 1982
M-mode contrast echocardiography in congenital heart disease
Echocardiography One. Ed Hunter S and Hall R J C
(Churchill Livingstone: Edinburgh)

Logan-Sinclair R B, Wong C M and Gibson D G 1981
Chemical application of amplitude processing of echocardiographic images
Br. Heart J. 45 621

Macartney F J, Smallhorn J F, Rees P E, Taylor J F N, de Leval M R and
Stark J 1983
Is cardiac catheterisation still essential to the diagnosis of congenital
heart disease?
Echocardiography Two, Ed by Hunter S and Hall R J C
(Churchill Livingstone: Edinburgh) to be published

Roelandt J, Meltzer R S, McGhie J and ten Cate F J 1982
Echocardiography of the cardiomyopathies
Echocardiography One, Ed Hunter S and Hall R J C
(Churchill Livingstone: Edinburgh)

Silverman N H and Snider A R 1982
Two-dimensional echocardiography - congenital heart disease
(Appleton - Century - Crofts: Connecticut)

Silverman N H, Snider A R and Gold J 1982
A segmental approach to the diagnosis of congenital heart disease: the
usefulness of two dimensional echocardiography.
Echocariography One, Ed Hunter S and Hall R
(Churchill Livingston: Edinburgh) 1982.

Smallhorn J F, Tommasini G, Anderson R H and Macartney F J 1982
Assessment of atrioventricular septal defects by two dimensional
echocardiography
Br.   Hear J. 47 109

Sutherland G R, Cottrell A J, Dias R C and Hunter S 1980
Rhabdomyoma of the interventricular septum in a neonate - two-dimensional
echocardiographic features
Eur.   Heart J.   1   461

Sutherland G R, Godman M J, Smallhorn J F, Guieteras P, Anderson R H and
Hunter S 1982
Ventricular septal defects.   Two-dimensional echocardiographic and
morphological correlations
Br.   Heart J.   47 316

Sutton M G St J, Sutton M St J, Oldershaw R, Sacchetti R, Paneth M,
Lennox S C, Gibson R V and Gibson D G 1981
Valve replacemnet without preoperative cardiac catheterisation
New England Journal of Medicine 305 1233

Imaging Techniques with Ultrasound

W N McDicken

Department of Medical Physics and Medical Engineering, Royal Infirmary, Edinburgh EH3 9YW

Abstract. In this introductory paper, points of basic principle have been emphasised if they are particularly relevant to cardiology or if they are somewhat neglected in the literature of the subject. The basic principles of ultrasonic imaging equipment are briefly described with consideration being given to the strengths and weaknesses of each type of unit. The applications of this equipment are found in the other ultrasonics contributions. The performance to be expected of those machines is briefly outlined. Possible improvements in cardiac imagers which can be expected in the near future are discussed. The way in which scanners can be used with other techniques are indicated, for example with Doppler blood flow measurements, needle and catheter guidance or contrast agents. Invasive scanners and three-dimensional scanners are also mentioned. Finally the question of safety is considered.

1. Introduction

Other papers in this section describe in detail ultrasonic techniques in cardiology namely Doppler flow measurement, wall motion recording, application of real-time scanners, tissue characterisation and clinical application. This paper provides an overview of diagnostic ultrasound technology, emphasising points which are particularly relevant to cardiology. Some aspects of the principles which are often neglected are discussed in detail. Finally a number of techniques are considered which have proven useful in other fields and which might have a place in cardiology. Two features of the ultrasonic method make it well suited to cardiac diagnosis namely the imaging of tissue motions and the measurement of blood flow.

2. Basic principles

The basic principles of diagnostic ultrasonic techniques are widely described in the literature (McDicken 1981, Wells 1977).

2.1 Beam shapes

All established techniques depend on the fact that directional beams of ultrasound can be generated with small transducers which can be held in the hand. This is somewhat surprising when the divergence of audible sound is considered. However, in diagnostic ultrasound high frequencies in the MHz range are employed, resulting in wavelengths which are much smaller than the diameter of the transducer crystal. Typically the wavelengths are less than 1 mm and the diameter of a transducer is around 20 wavelengths.   Diffraction effects are therefore less obvious and a directional beam is generated.

A simple description of a transmitted ultrasound beam usually presents it as a pencil shape of diameter roughly equal to the diameter of the transducer crystal.   More detailed plotting of the transmitted intensity pattern can be undertaken with a small point detector which is moved throughout the space in front of the transducer.   In diagnostic techniques the transducer is used both as a transmitter to generate the ultrasound and as a receiver to detect echoes.   The effective beam shape is therefore determined by both the transmitted intensity pattern and the reception sensitivity pattern   (Fig. 1).

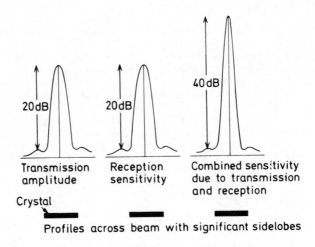

Fig. 1 The addition of transmission amplitude and sensitivity-amplitude profiles across a beam showing how their combination effectively narrows the beam.

This results in the effective beam width being narrower than might be expected from a typical transducer of diameter 15 mm.   There are two reasons for this effective beam narrowing.   First, the transmitted ultrasound pattern is most intense near the central axis of the beam   and second, the reception sensitivity is highest near the central axis. Structures are therefore more likely to be detected when they are close to the central axis.   The combined effect of transmission and reception patterns often produces a beam which is effectively 2 or 3 mm wide, particularly when weak reflectors are being detected.   It is therefore possible to depict small structures such as ducts and blood vessels within organs.   At present, resolution can be achieved adequate for visualisation of the major coronary arteries and improved resolution can be expected in the future.

2.2 Echoes from tissue

To produce echoes from structures within the body, a short pulse of ultrasound is transmitted through the tissues.

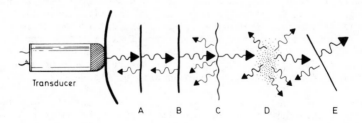

Fig. 2 Production of echoes at different types of tissue
boundaries.

The pulse is usually about 1 or 2 mm in length and consists of 2 or 3
pressure fluctuation cycles. Echoes are produced at regions where the
acoustic properties of the tissues alter e.g. the density or rigidity of
the tissue. Such regions range from large smooth tissue boundaries to
small cells. Care has to be taken when interpreting echoes resulting
from small scattering centres such as cells or organ parenchyma. (Fig.2).
Consider two point scatterers each of which produces an echo signal of
the shape shown in Fig. 3 a.

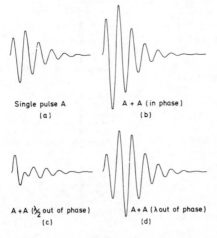

Single pulse A   A + A (in phase)
    (a)   (b)

A + A (½ out of phase)   A + A (λ out of phase)
    (c)   (d)

Fig. 3 The addition of echo pulses illustrating how the
result depends on their phase difference which is determined
by the separation of the targets producing the echoes.

If the scatterers are next to each other, there is no phase difference between the echoes so they add constructively, i.e. constructive interference occurs to produce a large echo (Fig. 3 b). If the scatterers are half of a wavelength ($\lambda/2$) apart, the echoes interfere destructively and produce a weak echo (Fig. 3 c). For a separation of λ, a strong echo signal is again produced. The size of the echo signal from a region of scattering centres, depends therefore on the distribution of the scatterers as well as their individual scattering properties (Morrison et al 1980). This makes it difficult to interpret exactly the echo magnitudes from within tissue structures like liver, blood or muscle. To obtain a reasonable measure of the reflectivity of tissues, the echo signals from the scatterers must be averaged over an area of tissue e.g. 2 cm^2.

The echo pattern in an image of organ tissue is an interference pattern and does not truly depict the tissue structure. The pattern is sometimes referred to as a speckle pattern. Since the speckle pattern does not depict tissue structure, the motion of the tissue does not produce a corresponding motion of the speckle pattern. Indeed the motion of the speckle pattern is usually completely unrelated to the tissue motion. The speckle pattern could move, for instance, more rapidly and in a different direction from the tissue. Detailed study of the motion of heart muscle must therefore be made with considerable care.

2.3 Focusing

With single crystal transducers, focusing is performed either by shaping the crystal or using a lens. The beam direction is altered by moving the whole transducer. Using a transducer consisting of several crystal elements, it is possible to perform focusing and beam deflection by wholly electronic means. A phased array scanner, common in cardiology, has a transducer constructed from several parallel crystal strips, e.g. 32, the complete transducer face being around 20 mm x 10 mm. Fig. 4 is a schematic representation of the mode of operation of this type of transducer. When the elements are excited simultaneously, the beam is emitted perpendicular to the crystal face (Fig. 4 a). With increasing delay of the excitation pulses from one crystal strip to the next, the beam is transmitted at an angle to the transducer axis (Fig. 4 b). To vary the angle, the delays are varied. The beam can therefore be steered rapidly through 90° without physically moving the transducer. Further adjustment of the delay pattern of the excitation pulses can result in a focused beam (Fig. 4c). Since reception is the converse of transmission, beam steering and focusing of the reception sensitivity

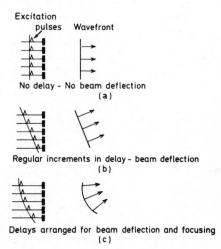

Excitation pulses   Wavefront

No delay - No beam deflection
(a)

Regular increments in delay - beam deflection
(b)

Delays arranged for beam deflection and focusing
(c)

Fig. 4 Ultrasound beam steering and focusing by varying the delay applied to each excitation signal.

zone is implemented by introducing appropriate delays to the echo signals detected by each crystal element.

It is worth noting that the electronic focusing with a phased array is partial since it is in the direction at right angles to the crystal strips. There is no focusing in the direction parallel to the strips. For complete focusing i.e. about the axis of the beam, a two-dimensional array is required. Arrays of this type are at an early stage of development. Complete electronic focusing can also be performed with an annular array transducer which consists of several (e.g. 10) concentric annular crystals. This type of array is being introduced to mechanical scanners which steer the beam by moving the transducer.

2.4 Ultrasound in tissue

The markedly different tissues and gas in the thorax pose large problems for the examination of the heart with ultrasound (Goss et al 1978). The acoustic properties of these materials are significantly different from each other (Table 1). An ultrasound beam is strongly attenuated in bone

Tissue	Ultrasonic properties		
	Attenuation (3 MHz) (thickness to half intensity)	Velocity	Acoustic impedance (density x velocity)
Blood	5.7 cm	1570 m/s	1.6×10^5 g/cm^{2}s
Muscle	0.5	1580	1.7×10^5
Bone	0.1	3500	7.8×10^5
Gas	0.1	330	0.0004×10^5
Liver	1.0	1550	1.6×10^5
Fat	1.7	1450	1.4×10^5
Soft tissue (average)	1.4	1540	1.6×10^5

Table 1.

but is transmitted readily through blood. Both bone and lung gas reflect ultrasound strongly since there is a large difference in their acoustic impedance from that of soft tissue. Indeed, gas acts as a complete barrier to ultrasound. Little information is available on cartilage. However, cartilage does appear to permit the passage of ultrasound without serious degradation of the beam.

Access to the heart with ultrasound is limited to windows determined by the acoustic properties of tissue and gas. Conventionally the heart is scanned from 2 or 3 rib spaces to the left of the sternum. Some access is also possible from above the rib cage, the suprasternal views. More recently views from below the rib cage have been used, the subxyphoid and apical views. The latter in fact allow considerable access to the heart. The soft bone of neonates and fetuses presents few problems for ultrasound so the heart is more accessible in these instances.

These access limitations have very significant implications for the design of equipment. Sector field-of-view instruments have proven to be the most successful as they make best use of the access windows. Access varies from patient to patient and this has a major bearing on the success of any examination.

3. Instrumentation

M-mode recordings of the motion of cardiac structures have been made for more than two decades.   The ultrasound beam is held fixed in a direction to intersect the cardiac structures of interest.   Pulses are regularly transmitted and each train of echo signals is recorded as spots on a line. These adjacent lines of echo spots build up to form the M-mode trace (Fig. 5).   A fibre-optic chart recorder is used for this purpose since it can handle the large number of fast signals in each echo train. The development of fibre-optic chart recorders was very significant in making the M-mode technique into a routine clinical tool.   It can also be noted from Fig. 5 that the beam direction may be slowly moved during an exam-ination so that the motions of neighbouring structures are recorded.

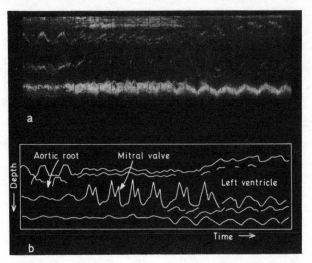

Fig. 5 M-mode strip chart record.   Initially the ultrasound beam was directed through the aortic root and then it was swept down past the mitral valve to the left ventricle.

Technical develop-ments over the last decade have largely been aimed at providing moving images of heart structures.   One method of imaging with ultrasound, the B-scan method, is long established.   The transducer, and hence its beam, is constrained to move in a single plane which is determined by the oper-ator.   The beam sweeps through a selected section of the body and for each beam direction a train of echoes is received.   Since the beam direction into the body is measured at each instant, each echo train is readily presented as a line of dots in the corresponding direction on the display screen to build up the image.   As the velocity of sound is high in tissue, approximately 1540 m/s, each echo train is received in a short time interval after the transmitted pulse is generated e.g. within 250 µs. One image, of say 100 lines, is then completed in 25ms, making it possible to produce 40 images per second i.e. a frame rate of 40/s.   Real-time imaging is the name given to techniques which produce many frames per second.   With real-time imaging the motion of heart valves and walls can be observed.   A second major benefit of real-time imaging is the ease with which the operator can scan through neighbouring image planes to find a structure of interest or to construct a mental three-dimensional image.   There are 5 basic approaches to the design of real-time imaging equipment.   These will now be briefly described and their advantages and disadvantages will be listed from the point of view of cardiology.

3.1 Mechanical oscillating transducer scanner

This type of scanner is particularly simple in that it is only necessary
to drive one transducer in an oscillating motion and to measure its
angular position at each instant (McDicken et al 1974a , Griffith and
Henry 1974). Several elegant designs have resulted in smooth running
devices (Fig. 6). Both the size of the field of view and the frame rate
are often restricted with this
approach e.g. a 70° sector and
a frame rate of 15/s. Since
only one transducer is required,
it is a practical proposition
to utilise a multi-crystal
annular array for complete
electronic focusing. Table
2 lists the advantages and
disadvantages of a mechanical
oscillator. The main dis-
advantage is that it is
necessary to stop the transducer in a selected position
to obtain a high quality M-
mode trace from a particular
region of the heart. On
balance, however, it can be
seen that this approach to
real-time imaging has much to
commend it.

3.2 Mechanical rotating transducer scanner

Another method of sweeping the
ultrasound beam quickly in a
real-time scanner is to mount
several transducers on a
rotating wheel (Barber et al
1974, Holm et al 1975). The
wheel is usually immersed in an
oil-filled plastic cylinder (Fig.
7) (Bow et al 1979). Each
transducer is activated when
its beam direction passes
through the field-of-view.
The plastic cylinder is
thin-walled at this position
so that transmission of
ultrasound into the patient
is accomplished with little
attenuation. The whole
transducer head is designed
to minimise spurious multiple
reflections in it. The field
of view is typically a 90°
sector and the frame rate is
variable up to 40/s.

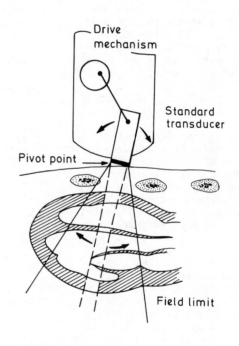

Fig. 6 Mechanical oscillator real-
time scanner.

Mechanical oscillator

Advantages

   Good beam shape
   Field of view - sector (60°)
   Small transducer assembly
   Complete electronic focusing
   Inexpensive
   Easy to alter ultrasound frequency

Disadvantages

Frame rate (up to 25/s)	
M-mode	stop transducer
	second transducer
Moving parts	

Table 2

It can be noted from Table 3 that the advantages of this design outweigh the disadvantages. As for the oscillating scanner, it is easy to incorporate standard single crystal transducers with good quality ultrasound beams. The potential for complete electronic focusing also exists with this unit. As for oscillating devices, the problems of wear of the moving parts have yet to be fully ascertained.

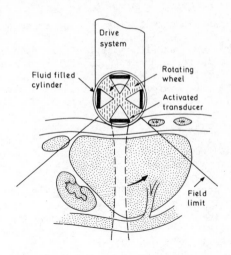

Fig. 7 Mechanical rotator real-time scanner.

3.3 Phased array (Electronic sector scanner)

It was noted earlier that an ultrasound beam can be steered using an array transducer without physically moving the transducer (Fig. 8) (Somer 1968). The performance of these devices has improved steadily over the last 10 years. Though their beam, and hence image quality, is somewhat inferior to devices using standard single crystal transducers and linear arrays, described in the next section, phased arrays have proven to be popular in cardiology due to the small size of the transducer assembly. Modern units have many crystal elements, e.g. 64, and are driven in a manner which improves their beam shapes e.g. the reduction of side-lobes by the use of apodisation which weights the contribution from each element. The phased array is also popular since several simultaneous M-mode traces can be recorded during imaging. Simultaneous M-mode recording is possible with electronic scanners, as distinct from mechanical scanners, since any beam direction can be selected for repeated examination during the scan sweep of the imaging mode. The advantages and disadvantages of phased arrays are shown in Table 4.

<u>Mechanical rotator</u>

Advantages

    Good beam shape
    Field of view - sector (90°)
    Small transducer assembly
    Frame rate (up to 40/s)
    Complete electronic focusing
    Inexpensive

Disadvantages

M-mode	stop transducer
	second transducer
Moving parts	

Table 3

3.4 Linear arrays

Fig. 9 is a schematic representation of a linear array imager (Bom et al 1971). The array consists of a large number of parallel strip crystal elements, e.g. 300 adjacent elements in a length of 15 cm. A beam is generated by exciting a group of elements simultaneously. To sweep the beam through the body, the group of elements is systematically changed after each cycle of transmission and reception. When linear arrays

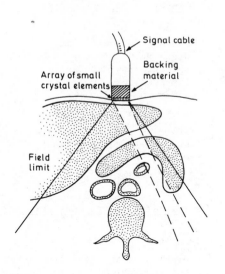

Fig. 8 Phased array real-time
scanner

Phased array

Advantages

Field of view - sector (90°)
Small transducer assembly
High frame rate (up to 70/s)
Several simultaneous M-modes
No moving parts

Disadvantages

Beam shape not optimum (side
   lobes)
Partial electronic focusing
Expensive
Low frequency of ultrasound

Table 4

were introduced they gave a major boost to real-time imaging.   These
devices are now primarily used in abdominal scanning.   However, they are
suited to paediatric heart imaging where attenuation from bone is not a
problem.   Table 5 lists the advantages and disadvantages.

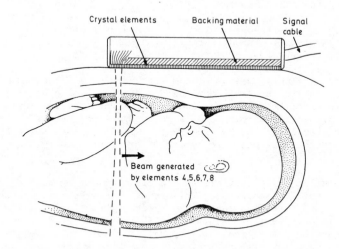

Fig. 9 Linear array real-time scanner.

3.5 Water-bath scanners

With any of the above scanners, it is possible to place a small water-
bath between the transducer and the patient's skin.   Structures close to
the skin surface, e.g. blood vessels, are then imaged more clearly as
they lie in a better focused region of the beam.   High frequency ultrasound, 5 to 10 MHz, may be employed since the desired depth of penetration

is usually less than 6 cm. Scanners which operate at high frequencies and are used to visualise superficial structures are often called 'small-part' scanners. They have potential for cardiac examinations in neonates. Table 6 gives a list of advantages and disadvantages for water-bath scanners. One unique advantage of water-bath scanners is that large aperture trans-ducers can be employed with a result-ing high quality of focused beam. On the other hand water-bath scanners may suffer from spurious signals as a result of multiple reflections in the water-bath.

It can be seen from this discussion that no scanner is perfect for all tasks. It is however relatively easy to choose an appropriate scanner for a particular clinical application.

4. Use of ultrasonic scanner

4.1 Resolution

In ultrasonic imaging the resolution attainable is always of importance. The resolution depends on a number of factors e.g. the ultrasonic pulse length and beam width. The differ-ences in reflectivity, i.e. the contrast, in the scanned tissues is also important. Finally, motion of the tissue is usually detrimental but in some circumstances small motions can provide averaging of the speckle echoes from within tissues and these improve the resolution. It is therefore almost impossible to make an accurate comprehensive state-ment as to the resolution to be expected. However, with 3 MHz pulsed ultrasound, it should be possible to depict structures down to 2 or 3 mm in size.

Temporal resolution may be defined as the minimum time between events for which they may both be observed. This resolution is determined by the frame rate. For heart scanning, frame rates higher than 25/s are desirable. To observe the most rapid motions of cardiac structures, i.e. the detailed actions of valves, it is usual to resort to M-mode recording where the echo sampling rate is typically more than 500/s.

4.2 Measurement

Since ultrasonic techniques essentially detect interfaces, measurement of dimensions is easily carried out. Individual frames are stored in a digital memory, allowing linear or area measurements to be performed. Volumes are calculated from a number of two-dimensional images and an appropriate formula. Table 7 gives an indication of the accuracies

Electronic linear array

Advantages

    Reasonable beam shape
    High frame rate (up to 70/s)
    Several simultaneous M-modes
    Inexpensive
    No moving parts

Disadvantages

    Field of view - rectangle
    Large transducer assembly
    Partial electronic focusing

Table 5

Water-bath scanner (Small parts scanner)

Advantages

    Highly focused beam from large
        transducer
    Complete electronic focusing
    Inexpensive

Disadvantages

    Field of view - trapezoid
    Large transducer assembly
    Frame rate (up to 25/s)
    M-mode   stop transducer
                second transducer
    Moving parts

Table 6

Measurement from real-time images (3 MHz ultrasound)

- dimensions measured $\pm$ 1 or 2 mm
- areas calculated $\pm$ 3%
- volumes calculated $\pm$ 10%
- echo amplitude $\pm$ 20%

Errors arise mainly from identification of boundaries or drop-out of echoes from parts of image.

Table 7

which are typical when structures are clearly and completely recorded.

4.3 Recording

A still photograph does little to portray the quality of a moving real-time image of the heart. There are a number of reasons for this, not all of which have been fully studied. Motion helps the observer to disregard spurious echoes. The eye is sensitive to moving edges and also integrates over a few frames, reducing the noise in the image. Anyone interested in heart imaging should therefore make a point of visiting an experienced operator who has an up-to-date machine. The recording techniques found in echocardiography are listed in Table 8. The video-tape recorder is the most popular for real-time imaging and the fibre-optic recorder for M-mode.

4.4 Machine tests

Tissue equivalent phantoms for testing ultrasonic imaging equipment are now available commercially. It has taken a number of years to devise media which mimic tissue realistically from an ultrasonic point of view (Madsen

Recording techniques

Frozen frame (ECG linked)
Video (tape or disc)
Digital disc
Cine film
Fibre-optic chart

Table 8

et al 1978, McCarty and Stewart 1982). The basic material is usually stabilised gelatin containing graphite particles. Low and high echogenic structures are incorporated as tests of sensitivity, nylon filaments are arranged to provide tests of spatial resolution. Such test phantoms can be used to check individual performance factors, but in routine clinical practice they are of most value in checking constancy of performance. Moving phantoms are being developed at present and will provide an improved check on real-time cardiac scanners.

5. Future developments in scanners

Although in many instances good ultrasonic images are produced, it is felt by many people that further improvement is desirable. It is interesting to try to identify the reasons for this and to see if improvements can be expected in the near future.

One problem at present is the difficulty in accurately compensating for attenuation of the ultrasound beam in the cardiac tissues. Blood has a low attenuation rate compared to muscle. The size of the chambers and the muscle thickness change throughout the heart cycle.

With simple controls on instruments, the operator fixes the rate of compensation with depth, i.e. the time gain compensation (TGC). This is at best an average compensation. It does not take into account either the different attenuation for each beam direction or the change in attenuation with the cardiac cycle. A technique which is beginning to be introduced is the use of automatic time gain compensation (ATGC) (McDicken et al 1974b). Here the machine detects echoes using no TGC or crudely set up TGC and derives a more. accurate TGC from this initial data. Since this automatic TGC is derived electronically, it can be performed rapidly and so vary with the beam direction and the phase of the heart cycle.

Resolution in ultrasonic images is directly related to ultrasonic frequency. With increasing frequency, it is possible to generate shorter pulses and narrower beams. Unfortunately attenuation increases with frequency. At present much of heart scanning is done at 3 MHz; however, calculations and tests with modern abdominal scanners show that adequate penetration can often be obtained at 5 MHz. Phased arrays are difficult to construct at 5 MHz due to the reduction in scale of the transducer head. No doubt this will be overcome in due course. More use of 5 MHz scanners is to be expected in the immediate future.

As noted earlier, phased arrays and linear arrays use partial electronic focusing. A few experimental two-dimensional arrays with complete electronic focusing have been developed. It would appear to be some time before such arrays will be commercially available. Hand-held mechanical scanners with complete electronic focusing using annular arrays are becoming commercially available.

In general, colour presentations have not proven popular in ultrasonic imaging since the images are noisy and a suitable method of using colour has not been found. However, in heart studies, colour imaging is being considered more seriously since it is felt that it can help to show the motion of walls more clearly and perhaps provide information on the reflecting properties of the muscle tissue.

6. Ultrasonic imaging plus Doppler techniques

One of the attractions of ultrasonic imaging techniques is that it is easy to link them with other methods. A powerful combination is a real-time scanner to depict cardiac structures plus a Doppler probe to detect blood flow at particular sites in the heart (Fig. 10) (Baker et al 1977, Atkinson and Woodcock 1982). The measurement of a blood vessel diameter from the image and blood velocity information from the Doppler instrument give the necessary data for the quantification of blood flow. This technique and its refinement is discussed in a later paper. Usually pulsed wave (PW) ultrasound is used, but continuous wave (CW) devices are also employed.

Rather than have the Doppler probe attached to the scanner as shown in Fig. 10, it is also common to use one of the probes in the scanner head to fulfil a second role as the Doppler probe. Fig. 11 shows the display of a combined imager and Doppler unit applied to measure flow in the descending aorta. The position of the sample volume of the Doppler unit is indicated by the short line in the blood vessel.

The detection of blood flow at sites within organs and blood vessels means that it is possible to build up an image depicting regions of blood flow. The velocity at each site can be presented using a colour code related to velocity. This type of imaging is intrinsically slower than pulsed-echo imaging since a low frequency signal has to be measured at

each site. Doppler signals are in
the audio frequency range. To date
Doppler imaging in the heart has
only been carried out to a limited
extent.

7. Miscellaneous ultrasonic techniques

The technology of ultrasonics is
flexible and relatively inexpensive. This opens up a wide
range of applications.

7.1 Guided needles and catheters

One popular technique is to use
an ultrasonic imager to guide a
biopsy needle or catheter to a
selected location in the body
(Holm et al 1978). Tissue can
then be extracted or a
contrast agent injected.
The technique is not
widely used in cardio-
logy at present.

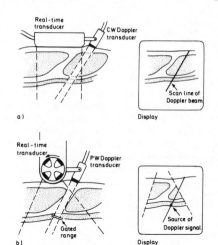

Fig. 10 Externally linked real-time
scanners and Doppler transducers.

7.2 Contrast agents

Contrast media for
cardiology are liquids
such as dextrose,
saline or indocyanine
green which have micro-
bubbles suspended in
them (Gramiak et al
1969, Meltzer and
Roelandt 1982). These
contrast liquids have
been very profitably
employed to identify
cardiac structures,
particularly in M-
mode work, and to
detect shunts between
chambers in the heart.

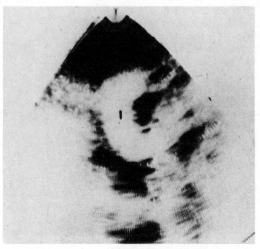

Fig. 11 The descending aorta with the Doppler
sample volume located centrally.

Contrast agents are now being studied thoroughly
to make the effect more reproducible and to quantify their motion.

7.3 Invasive ultrasonics

Although ultrasonic methods are normally described as non-invasive, the
quality of the results now justifies using them in an invasive role. Real-
time scanners have been constructed for prostate scanning via the rectum
and for insertion into the bladder for tumour staging. Ultrasonic
imagers have been added to the end of endoscopes for examining the wall of
the stomach. Experimental imaging and Doppler instruments have been put
into the oesophagus for studying the heart without interference from ribs

or lung gas.   Instruments are also employed during surgery.

7.4 Three-dimensional imaging

Just as an ultrasound beam can be made to scan in 2 dimensions and echoes
collected from each beam direction, it can be made to scan in 3 dimensions.
The main problem is to display the 3D information in a suitable manner.
Anterior echo signals obscure posterior ones in most displays when the
echo density is high.   In cardiology this may be less of a difficulty
than in abdominal work as well defined heart chambers may be identified.
Some laboratory systems have been described for 3D scanning (Matsumoto et
al 1977).   It is worth remembering however that searching with a conventional real-time scanner effectively results in a 3D study of the heart.
In other fields the interest in 3D imaging has been limited.

8. Safety

A large number of techniques exist in the ultrasonics laboratory which
could find application in the long term in cardiology.   Ultrasonic beams
and signals are very amenable to manipulation.   Figure 12 shows that
there is a reasonable
safety margin with the
established techniques
which propagate short
pulses or low power
continuous wave ultra-
sound (Kremkau 1980).
Nevertheless,as new
techniques are developed
they will have to be
examined carefully for
possible hazards.
Blood in motion is
known to be a medium in
which cavitation bubbles
are easily generated.
These bubbles can rupture
cells.

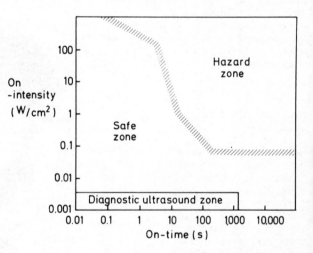

9. Conclusions

Ultrasonic techniques   Fig. 12 The division of hazard and safety zones
for cardiology are far   for ultrasonic exposures at diagnostic
from being fully   frequencies.
developed and are
well suited to the investigation of the heart.   When they are compared
with other physical methods it is useful to list their advantages and
disadvantages (Table 9).

The first two advantages arise from the fact that ultrasonic information
can be collected and processed quickly.   Echo information to produce one
image is collected within 40 ms and blood flow velocity spectra can be
generated at intervals of less than 10 ms.   The non-invasive nature and
the duration of an examination (e.g. 20 min) make it highly practical as
a routine tool.   Although access to the heart can be difficult, useful
diagnostic information can be obtained in most cases.   Future developments should reduce the other disadvantages.

Ultrasonic techniques in cardiology

Advantages

Images of moving tissues
Blood flow detection at specific sites
Measurements of dimensions
Non-invasive and non-hazardous
Reasonably quick examination

Disadvantages

Access to heart may be difficult in
some cases
Results only partially quantitative
at present
Image quality could be better
Little information about state of
muscle

Table 9

10. References

Atkinson P and Woodcock J P 1982 Doppler Ultrasound and its use in
Clinical Measurement (London, Academic Press)
Baker D W, Rubenstein S A and Lorch G S 1977 Am. J. Med. 63 69-80
Barber F E, Baker D W and Strandness Jr D E et al 1974 IEEE Ultrasonics
Sym. Proc. 744-8
Bom, N, Lancee C T, Honkoop J et al 1971 Biomed. Eng. 6 500-8
Bow C R, McDicken W N and Anderson T et al 1979 Br. J. Radiol. 52 29-33
*Chang S 1976 M-Mode Echocardiographic Techniques and Pattern Recognition
(Philadelphia, Lea and Febiger)
*Feigenbaum H 1981 Echocardiography 3rd Ed. (Philadelphia, Lea and
Febiger)
Goss S A, Johnston R L and Dunn F 1978 J. Acoust. Soc. Am. 64 423-57
Gramiak R, Shah B M and Kramer D H 1969 Radiology 92 939-48
Griffith J M and Henry W L 1974 Circulation 49 1147-52
Holm H H, Kristensen J K, Pedersen J F and Hancke S 1975 Ultrasound
Med. Biol. 2 19-23
Holm H H and Gammelgard J 1978 Ultrasonically guided biopsy in malignant
disease in Hill C R, McCready V R, Cosgrove D O (eds) 1978 Ultrasound
in Tumour Diagnosis (Tunbridge Wells, Pitman)
*Hussey M 1975 Diagnostic Ultrasound (Glasgow, Blackie)
Kremkau F W 1980 Diagnostic Ultrasound (New York, Grune and Stratton)
pp 132-9
McCarty K and Stewart W 1982 Ultrasound Med. Biol. 8 393-401
McDicken W N, Bruff K and Paton J 1974a Ultrasonics 12 269-72
McDicken W N, Evans D H and Robertson D A R 1974b Ultrasonics 12 173-6
McDicken W N 1981 Diagnostic Ultrasonics: Principles and Use of
Instruments 2nd Ed (New York, Wiley)
Madsen E L, Zagzebski J A, Banjavie R A et al 1978 Med. Phys. 5 391-4
Matsumoto M, Matsuo H, Kitabatake A et al 1977 Ultrasound Med. Biol. 3
168-78
Meltzer R and Roelandt J 1982 Contrast Echocardiography (The Hague,
Martinus Nijhoff Publishers)
Morrison D, McDicken N and Wild R 1980 Appl. Radiol. 9 109-12
Reneman R S 1974 Cardiovascular Applications of Ultrasound (Amsterdam,
Excerpta Medica/North Holland)
Somer J C 1968 Ultrasonics 6 153-9

*Thijssen J M (ed) 1980 Ultrasonic Tissue Characterisation: Clinical
   achievements and technological potentials (The Netherlands,
   Stafleu's Scientific Publishing Company)
 Wells P N T 1977 Biomedical Ultrasonics (London, Academic Press)
*Wells P N T and Ziskin M C 1981 New Techniques and Instrumentation in
   Ultrasonography (Edinburgh, Churchill Livingstone)

* Not in text but included as suggested further reading.

Real-Time Cardiac Imaging

by N. Bom and H. Rijsterborgh

Thoraxcenter,Erasmus University Rotterdam and Interuniversity Cardiology
Institute of the Netherlands.

1. Introduction

The subject of real-time cardiac imaging has many aspects. These range
from automation to possibilities of new machines. In this paper only four
topics will be discussed. The first topic concerns activities to
quantitate two-dimensional left ventricular images by contour
enhancement.
It is difficult to derive ventricular contours in any repeatable way
from still frames. Therefore, in 1979, we developed an interactive
processing computer system, based on sequential frame information. The
method is described by Vogel et al (1979). As a result,in a semi-
automatic way, the full two-dimensional real-time image could be
reconstructed. The reconstructed contour can be presented in motion and
can be used for quantitative analysis. More recently a variety of contour
enhancement techniques have been described by Meerbaum et al. (1982).
These methods are based on temporal as well as spatial averaging
techniques. The data is obtained by direct digitization of the real-time
cardiac echo image.

It proved possible to derive "a contour". However, in our opinion it
seemed questionable whether it was allowable to use such quantitative
information for clinical evaluation of a patient's left ventricular
parameters when derived with similar techniques.

We therefore carefully studied inter-observer variability as well as
intra-observer variability and beat-to-beat variation on quantitative
data derived by contour methods from the left ventricle. It appeared that
great care is needed when using such information and that
present methods are far from being useful in routine applications.

A number of problems is caused by the still poor quality of echo images
as obtained from the heart. It is well known that transducers are of
major importance in the final echo image quality. The importance of
transducers in real-time cardiac imaging is the second topic in this
paper. It seems that much effort should be put into improvement of the
transducer sensitivity, bandwidth, as well as suppression of echoes
that do not arise from the transducer main axis.

With present echo imaging systems we   show the geometry of structures.
With exception of the Doppler method, no blood can be visualized. The
third topic is contrast echocardiography. This is a technique of
injecting an echo-producing biologically compatible solution into the
blood stream which reveals intra-cardiac bloodflow patterns by the
resulting cloud of echoes. This may be an alternative method to better
delineate cardiac contours better, but it is particularly useful in the
study of the haemodynamics of the heart such as in cases of shunts.

A fourth and more futuristic topic will be described at the end of this
paper. The heart has been imaged so far with the so-called "simple scan".
This means that any part of the cardiac tissue is only insonified from
one single direction. With the oncoming real-time compound systems it now
becomes possible to insonify the heart, in real time, from more than one
direction. A very first result of this approach shows that insonification
from more than one direction may be advantageous for image information.
The necessarily larger transducer does, however, put some limitations on
directional capabilities.

2. Quantitative information from cardiac contours

Clinical experience with video recordings has shown that a recording period
of several cardiac cycles and a recording speed of fifty images per
second is sufficient to obtain the necessary visual information. This may
be the basis of contour analysis. Two methods have been developed for
storage of analogue echo data in the computer system.
First there is the on-line digitization. This method consists of a fast
analogue-to-digital conversion as the two-dimensional images are
digitized on-line during the clinical investigation. The enormous data
rate which is required limits severely the selection of appropriate
information since the storage capacity only allows storage of a limited
number of cardiac cycles. The method described by Vogel et al (1979) is
based on reconstruction of two-dimensional images from successive lines
which are presented as M-mode. The operator selects the required
structure in the first M-mode (say corresponding to the top of the two-
dimensional image) and traces this with a light pen. On the next M-mode
in sequence, the computer uses the traced line as a first approximation
in its search for the structure. The new line is then displayed to the
operator who may accept or may correct the line using the light pen. The
combination of M-mode information is then used to derive the contour of
the two-dimensional image. This may be presented in motion and can be
used for further quantitative analysis. The strength of this method
is that reconstruction from M-mode allows the operator to integrate
information over a number of beats.
It proved to be possible to reconstruct in the above described way the
contours of, for instance, the endocardial surface of the left ventricle.
It proved unfortunately to be a quite lengthy procedure which was
be impractical for routine applications.

A second method for digitization is based on images preserved as video
recordings. Useful images for processing are selected from the complete
video recordings of the patient. This requires a real-time digitizer for
digitization into a video scanned memory. Processing starts with
automatic determination of maximum (white) and minimum (black) intensity
in the grey scale images. The resulting intensity range is divided into
sixteen digitizing levels. For a standard echocardiogram this division is
based on equidistant levels. With this method it became possible to

introduce an interactive technique based on segmentation of cardiac
structures in a series of one hundred successive images.

In addition the question arose of   how reliable quantification from two-
dimensional echocardiographic images really is.   In the recent literature
many reports can be found describing the possibility of extracting
quantitative information on local and global parameters of left
ventricular function from two-dimensional echocardiographic images. See
for example Folland et al (1979). The local parameters of left
ventricular function are local wall thickness or wall thickening and wall
motion, whereas the global parameters are instantaneous volume, stroke
volume, cardiac output and ejection fraction. Since two-dimensional
echocardiography can only provide cross-sectional views of the ventricle,
only local information can be extracted directly from the images. Usually
this local information is extrapolated to regional or segmental
information. Global parameters of left ventricular function are estimated
by integrating low quality information from multiple cross-sectional
views, making use of mathematical models of the left ventricle. With the
aid of an image processing system, a semi-automatic frame-by-frame
analysis was performed on sequences of two-dimensional echocardiographic
images recorded on video tape. Studies were made on a set of twenty
clinically normal subjects to determine average values for the
local parameters, wall motion and wall thickening. Using the same group of
subjects, the variability of the measurements was assessed. The two-
dimensional images, enabling optimal visualization of the left ventricle,

PSSAX-M   PSSAX-P

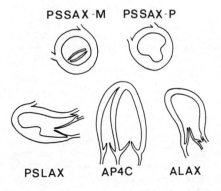

PSLAX   AP4C   ALAX

Figure 1.
The two short-axis and three long-axis views studied in the clinical
examination. (PSLAX = Parasternal long-axis view, PSSAX-M = Parasternal
short-axis view at mitral level, PSSAX-P = Parasternal short-axis view at
papillary level, AP4C = Apical four-chamber view, ALAX = Apical long-axis
view).
(Courtesy O. Bastiaans).

were obtained in five standard planes. The planes have been indicated in
figure 1. With the two-dimensional real-time images in mind, a stop
frame video and light pen technique was used for interactive
determination of muscular outlines on end-diastolic and end-systolic
images. This was used to quantify the local parameters from two-
dimensional images. A radial coordinate system was used for the
measurements since the short-axis views normally show a circular outline.
The center of this coordinate system was fixed at the geometrical center
of the endocardial outline in end-diastole. Results of the measurements
are presented as a function of position within the two-dimensional image
(see for example figure 2). In the short-axis views, zero degree is the
lateral wall and the polar angle increases counterclockwise. Wall
thickness as function of angle could be measured by sampling the outline.
Wall thickening could then be computed from wall thickness at end-
diastolic and end-systolic measurements.

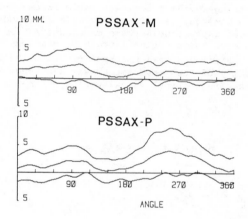

Figure 2.
The standard deviation of variability in measurement of wall thickening
expressed in mm. These values were calculated from the differences in wall
thickening as found by two independent observers. The middle curve shows
the average amplitude. The upper and lower curve delineate the range of
plus or minus one standard deviation.
(Courtesy O. Bastiaans)

Our interest was the random error and bias in the measurements, and the
derived global parameters. The outcome of the second measurement rarely
equals that of the first and the differences in bias and random error can
be computed from paired measurements. An accurate separation of bias and
random error can only be carried out if a sufficient number of
measurements are performed. In clinical research this requirement cannot
always be met. In the study described by Bastiaans et al (1981) the two
sources of error could not be studied separately and therefore only the
variability was assessed. Possible causes of this variability are:

- Limitations in resolution for digitization of outlines;
- Limitations in operator accuracy in defining the outlines;
- Changes in operator interpretation in defining the outlines;
- Limitations of operator accuracy in defining the same plane;
- Changes in operator interpretation in finding the same plane;
- Differences of interpretation by different observers.

In four separate experiments with different observers, inter-observer variability and intra-observer variability could be derived: the variability of the analysis methods could be demonstrated. The study also included the beat-to-beat variation.

Since the spread in measured wall motion and wall thickening between normal subjects is large, and since the inter-observer variability in these measurements appeared to be of the same magnitude as the measured values, it can be concluded that quantitative left ventricular analysis from two-dimensional echocardiography as described in the paper referred to, will not yield acceptable results for individual subjects. This study, which was carried out in our laboratory, indicates that care is needed when using derived quantitative information.

3. Transducers

It is well known that good transducers are of main importance in order to obtain high quality images. In real-time two-dimensional imaging of the heart, two transducer shapes are currently used. There are the disc shaped transuducer (fig. 3a) and the rectangular shaped transducer (fig. 3b). The disc shaped transducer is often used in various mechanical scanners. The rectangular transducer is the basis of the phased array sector scanners. It is well known that the directivity pattern of a square aperture has many "side lobes" which will cause noise due to echoes which are off the main axis. A calculation of the far field directivity pattern of a square aperture is presented in figure 4. Improvement can be obtained when focusing in one plane is introduced. This becomes possible when electronic delay lines are used. An example is given in figure 5, which shows the far field directivity pattern of a focused 12-element phased array with an array width of 24 mm, an array height of 10 mm and a frequency of 3.12 MHz. The two-dimensional echo sensitivity distribution in a logarithmic brightness display in a plane perpendicular to the acousitic axis at 80 mm actual distance is shown. Apparently a good improvement can be obtained.

Figures 3d and 3e show more futuristic approaches. A mosaic transducer might improve the resolution further, since lateral resolution in the plane perpendicular to the scanning plane can be obtained. An annular array transducer will yield further advantages since it combines good focusing capability with a suppression of side lobes due to its disc shaped geometry. A disadvantage would be the need for mechanical steering when a sector scan is required. Although it would require mechanical steering, it seems that a lot of effort is being put into development of new annular array transducers. However, the high flexibility of electronically steered rectangular shaped transducers is a great advantage. In addition no need for any mechanical steering device exists. With increased knowledge of beam pattern synthesis and suppression of off axis echoes it seems that the future lies with the electronically steered systems.

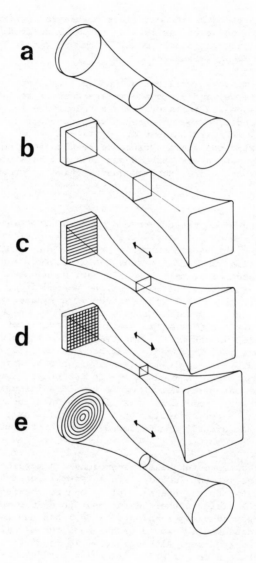

Figure 3.
Various basic transducer shapes as presently (and possibly in future)
used in real-time cardiac imaging.

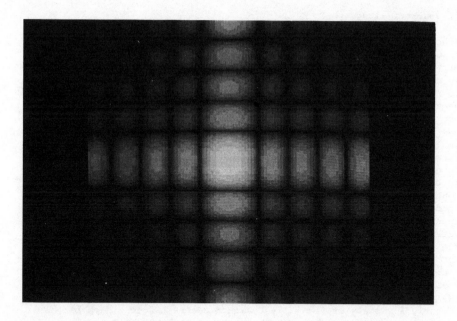

Figure 4.
Far field directivity pattern of a square aperture as calculated in the
so-called "C-scan" plane. Logarithmic brightness representation of echo
sensitivity in 16 grey levels. (Courtesy L. v.d. Wal).

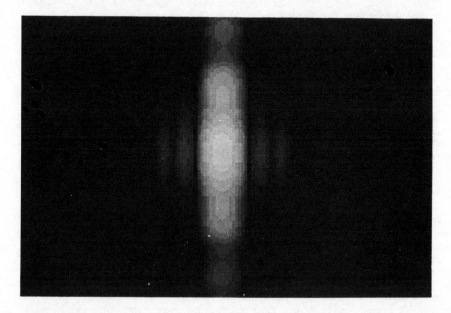

Figure 5.
Calculated far field directivity pattern in a "C-plane" with a focused
multiple-element rectangular transducer.

4. Contrast echography

Echocardiography allows us to differentiate cardiac structures from
bloodfilled cavities without use of contrast materials and is a highly
effective method for the study of cardiac anatomy and function. Doppler
is a method that derives the velocity of particles by measuring changes
in echo frequency. Since Doppler is used to "look" at blood, and blood is
usually not seen by ordinary echo instruments, it follows that Doppler
machines must be much more sensitive. A variety of contrast techniques
has been introduced to opacify the blood. The contrast agent may be
injected through, for instance, an 18 gauge needle positioned in a basilic
vein. Contrast echocardiological studies can be carried out in a routine
laboratory with ambulatory patients. It does not require anything more
intricate than a needle and a push injection of saline. A number of
contrast agents are available. Any biological compatible solution can be
used to deliver microbubbles present in the injectate and/or injecting
apparatus into the heart. The normal solutions include dextrose 5% in
water or saline. These are the currently most employed contrast agents
due to their lack of toxicity, their cheapness and the availability. In
most patients these solutions will yield adequate contrast effect after
either peripheral or central injection. In a recent review article by
Roelandt (1982) the present status of contrast echocardiography has been
fully described.
Recently a variety of specially designed contrast agents have become
available (Tickner, 1981). Microbubbles of carbondioxide
can be encapsulated in biologically compatible substances such as
gelatine and polysaccharides. The coating determines the life span and
course of the bubble in the blood stream. They can be made small enough
to pass the capillary bed. The large variability in obtaining adequate
contrast effect during routine studies remains one of the main problems
to be solved before the technique will gain wide-spread application.
Major applications of contrast echocardiography include structure
identification, diagnosis of shunts, identification of complex congenital
heart diseases and valvular insufficiency. Study of flow patterns and
possibilities of improved identification of left ventricular boundaries
may be further applications of contrast echocardiography. It seems a
rapidly developing field and will undoubtedly play an increasing role in
the daily practice of cardiology in future. Only when a quantifiable and
reliable non-toxic agent   is   found which is able to pass the lung, will
a definite break through appear. This is because one of the severe
limitations of echo contrast techniques is that the contrast can only
easily be provoked in the right ventricular cavities. For left
ventricular injection a catheter must be used.

5. Real-time compound scanning

So far only a simple scan of the heart can be obtained with real-time
techniques. This means that any part of the tissue is insonified by
ultrasound rays in one direction only. Therefore the number of drop-outs
is still quite high and it always remains difficult to view the apical
structures. With the introduction of a combination of linear arrays and
electronic sector scanners the so-called real-time compound scanning has
become available. It is now possible to integrate into a number of
sequential frames information from sector scanners from more than one
entry point. Thus it becomes possible to view the heart from more than
one direction and combine the images at appropriate real-time speed. It
is as if more than one search light is looking at the heart from a

variety of directions. Recently this method has been tried in only one
case for cardiac observation, but no information is yet available as
to the aiming problems of the larger transducer which is the basis of
"two search lights". (Ligtvoet and Eversdijk 1981).
It does seem, however, a first approach to obtaining information from the
heart from more directions and in more than one cross-sectional plane.
The future will reveal its importance.

6. Conclusion

Presently many studies are carried out in research laboratories to
improve the cardiac real-time image and/or the information derived from
its parameters. It appears that the quantitative contour approach is in
its infancy and not yet reliable. Additional information on delineation
of structures as well as haemodynamic information can be obtained with
contrast techniques. More effort should be put into transducer
development to improve the basis for all echo information, the
cardiac image.

References

Bastiaans O L , Meltzer R S et al 1981 Quantification from two-
    dimensional echocardiographic images. In: Rijsterborgh H (ed.)
    Echocardiology 131 - 143 Martinus Nijhoff Publishers, The Hague.
Folland E D, Parisi A F et al 1979 Assessment of left ventricular
    ejection fraction and volumes by real-time two-dimensional
    echocardiography. Circulation 60 No. 4 760-6
Ligtvoet C M, Eversdijk C H 1981 Real-time compound scanning In: Kurjak
    A and Kratochwil A (eds.) Real time Advances in Ultrasound Diagnosis 3
    51-55 Excerpta Medica, Amsterdam-Oxford-Princeton.
Meerbaum S, Garcia E et al 1982 Quantification of cardiac function by
    computerized two-dimensional echocardiography. In: Hanrath P and
    Bleifeld W (eds.) Cardiovascular diagnosis by Ultrasound 47-55.
    Martinus Nijhoff Publishers, The Hague.
Roelandt J 1982 (in press) Contrast Echocardiography. Ultrasound in Med
    & Biol 8.
Tickner E G 1981 Precision microbubbles for right side intracardiac
    pressure and flow measurements. In: Rijsterborgh H (ed.) Echocardiology
    461-472. Martinus Nijhoff Publishers, The Hague.
Vogel J A, Bastiaans O L et al 1979 Structure recognition and data
    extraction in two-dimensional echocardiography In: Lancee (ed.)
    Echocardiology 457-467. Martinus Nijhoff Publishers, The Hague.

M-Mode Echocardiography in the Study of Left Ventricular Function

D G Gibson

Cardiac Department, Brompton Hospital, Fulham Road, London SW3 6HP

Ultrasound has been widely used in cardiology to study the position, and particularly the motion of structures within the heart. Unlike its application in other branches of medicine, relatively few attempts have been made to characterise the structural echoes themselves. Over the past few years, two-dimensional echocardiography has attracted considerable interest in view of its ability to give a comprehensive view of cardiac anatomy from a variety of transducer positions. This ability has proved particularly valuable in the study of patients with complex congenital heart disease, and also left ventricular function in patients with coronary artery disease. The technique has also been used by numerous workers to estimate left ventricular volumes and ejection fraction. Although significant correlation can be established, the 95% confidence limits are wide, being of the order of 40-80 ml for ventricular volume and 10-20% for ejection francion (1,2), thus making the method of little value in individual cases, particularly for the detailed analysis of ventricular function or for documentation of changes due to drug administration or other manoeuvres. It is against this background that the possible place of M-mode echocardiography should be reconsidered.

When the technique was first introduced, M-mode echocardiograms were recorded 'blind', so the operator never knew the exact relation between the position of the ultrasound beam and that of the ventricle as a whole, a series of intracardiac landmarks being used. However, this approach is no longer necessary. The position at which the measurements are to be made is first localised from a two-dimensional display; with a phased array system, a simultaneous M-mode can be recorded and, with a mechanical system, the crystal is arrested in the required position. This development has circumvented the major drawback of M-mode echocardiography. Of particular value for analysis of intracardiac motion is a repetition rate of 1000/s compared with 30/s or even less for apical views achieved with two-dimensional systems. The high repetition rate is associated with greatly improved endocardial visualisation. The dynamic range of instruments has greatly increased, so that endo- and epicardial echoes can be recorded simultaneously. The latter can also be separated from the much more intense parietal pericardial echoes, so that more reliable estimates of regional wall thickness and dynamics are possible than with any other currently available method.

M-mode estimates of left ventricular transverse dimension have been widely studied. They correlate closely with minor dimension measured by angiography, with reproducibility of 2-3 mm (3,4). They can thus be used to document the effects of drugs or other physiological manoeuvres. Unlike angiography, M-mode echocardiography defines the position of the endocardium clearly at end-systole, so that it is possible to assess the degree of shortening of the minor dimension. This is remarkable, being between 25 and 40% in the normal. Using a combination of M-mode and two-dimensional echocardiography, it is possible to map the posterior wall of the left ventricle systematically, and to demonstrate regional differences in the degree of thickening which can be correlated with ventricular fibre architecture (5).

M-mode echocardiograms can be digitised in order to take advantage of the rapid repetition rate. This may be done automatically or manually (6). It is thus possible to obtain continuous traces of cavity dimension or wall thickness along with peak systolic and diastolic rates of change (Figure 1). These values have been validated by comparison with

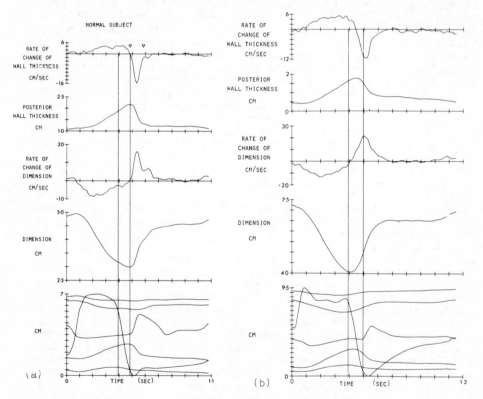

Figure 1.   (a)   Digitised M-mode echocardiogram from normal subject. Original digitised data are shown in lowest panel, and above, LV dimension, rate of change of dimension, wall thickness and (top), rate of change of wall thickness. The two vertical lines represent the timing of A2 and mitral valve opening. (b) Digitised M-mode echocardiogram from a patient with coronary artery disease. Layout as part (a). Note that there has been a significant increase in cavity dimension, and a fall in wall thickness during the period of isovolumic relaxation.

angiography (7). Finally, additional information can be recorded on M-mode records such as a mitral echogram, a phonocardiogram or a pulse tracing, and interrelations between various events in the cardiac cycle studied in considerable detail.

As an example, the use of this approach to the study of diastole will be considered (8). Isovolumic relaxation time can be estimated as the time interval between A2, the onset of the first high frequency vibration of the aortic component of the second heart sound, and the onset of mitral valve opening, determined from the mitral echogram. The former can be confirmed from its relation to the aortic echogram. Normal isovolumic relaxation time is approximately 60 + 10 ms (9), but is prolonged in left ventricular disease of all types, particularly left ventricular hypertrophy. By contrast, it is shortened when left ventricular end-diastolic pressure is raised, and may be zero when end-diastolic pressure is above 30 mmHg (10). Isovolumic relaxation time shortens with isometric exercise and lengthens with TNT administration in patients with coronary artery disease.

Following mitral valve opening, dimension increases rapidly, reaching a peak value of 10-20 cm/s (6). This is accompanied by thinning of the posterior wall at 15-25 cm/s, a rate very much more rapid than that of thickening during systole (11). This phase of rapid filling lasts 120-200 ms, and dimension then remains virtually constant in the normal subject until the onset of left atrial systole. This pattern of wall motion is lost, not only in patients with mechanical obstruction to inflow due, for example, to mitral stenosis, but also in those with left ventricular hypertrophy (12). Here, peak rates of dimension increase and of wall thinning are low, and the difference between the early phase of rapid filling and diastasis is obliterated. These changes can be used to assess the severity of the physiological disturbance caused by mitral stenosis, thus avoiding the need for cardiac catheterisation in many cases (13). Diastolic abnormalities are present in both primary and secondary left ventricular hypertrophy and persist when the underlying cause, such as aortic stenosis, is corrected, even though the left ventricular muscle mass falls. In these circumstances, therefore, they probably represent the presence of an irreversible change in myocardial function.

M-mode echocardiography has also been used to establish a series of well-defined relations between left ventricular wall motion and other events in the cardiac cycle which are present in normals, but which are very frequently lost in disease. An example is shown in Figure 1(b). Here there has been a significant increase in left ventricular dimension during isovolumic relaxation, showing that cavity shape must have changed. This pattern of motion is particularly common in patients with coronary artery disease, and appears to result from incoordination in the onset of relaxation. A second example is the relation between changes in left ventricular dimension and pressure. Normally, no significant dimension change occurs during the time of inscription of the upstroke or downstroke of the pressure pulse. This can be documented by construction of a pressure dimension loop which, in normal subjects, is rectangular (14), a configuration that has physical significance as the condition of optimal energy transfer from myocardium to the circulation (Figure 2). In patients with coronary artery disease the loop is distorted, mainly by abnormal dimension changes during the two isovolumic periods, rather than by abnormal pressure changes during ejection or filling. This leads to

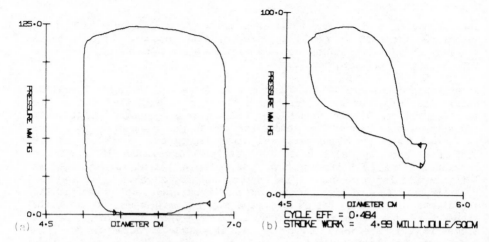

Figure 2.   (a) Pressure-dimension loop from a normal subject. Note the rectangular configuration.   (b) Pressure-dimension loop from a patient with coronary artery disease. Note that the loop is distorted, with reduction in cycle efficiency to 48% (normal; greater than 80%).

striking distortion of the loop and thus to loss of mechanical efficiency of energy transfer, regardless of the function of the myocardium itself. This process may affect areas of the ventricle well away from the site of the primary ischaemic process, indicating that these abnormalities of wall motion in patients with coronary artery disease are generalised, involving the greater part of the left ventricle. M-mode echocardiography has proved a particularly suitable method for detecting them, with its high repetition rate and excellent definition of endocardium in comparison with two - dimensional echocardiography. Their detection in patients with hypertension has clear clinical significance in that their presence is closely related to that of coronary artery disease which may be clinically silent (15).

M-mode and two-dimensional echocardiography are thus complementary. In view of constraints of path length and the velocity of sound, it is unlikely that the frame rate of two - dimensional echocardiographic apparatus will be increased as long as 100 lines are required for a single image. However, repetition rate can be increased if the line density is reduced, and we have modified a phased array system to give 40 scan lines per image (16). The information is presented not as a two-dimensional image, but as 40 simultaneous M-mode displays, scanning the heartfrom apex to base.. These M-mode records are then digitised and the resulting information can then be presented as an isometric display, or used to reconstruct the original image. Examples are shown in Figure 3.

One of the major achievements of echocardiography has been its ability to document the motion of intracardiac structures, using the M-mode technique. This has, to some extent, been lost sight of in the current preoccupation with two-dimensional systems which give an output that is much more easily assimilated in comparison with the more abstract M-mode records. However, these two techniques can now be used together in a variety of ways, allowing the unique physiological information obtained by M-mode to be added to the anatomical approach provided by two-dimensional systems.

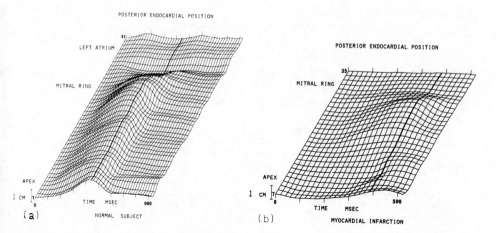

POSTERIOR ENDOCARDIAL POSITION

LEFT ATRIUM

MITRAL RING

APEX

1 CM

TIME   MSEC   900

(a)   NORMAL SUBJECT

POSTERIOR ENDOCARDIAL POSITION

MITRAL RING

APEX

1 CM

TIME   MSEC   500

(b)   MYOCARDIAL INFARCTION

Figure 3. (a) Multiple M-mode display of posterior endocardial position
from a normal subject. Each horizontal line represents the motion of
posterior wall endocardium during the cardiac cycle. The position of each
plot in the cavity is shown on the left of the display. Note the
coordinate pattern of wall motion. (b) Multiple M-mode display from a
patient with coronary artery disease. Note the abnormal pattern of
endocardial motion towards the apex.

References

1. Folland E D, Parisi A F, Moynihan P F, Jones D R, Feldman C L and
Tow D E 1979   Assessment of left ventricular ejection fraction and
volumes by real-time two-dimensional echocardiography. A comparison of
cineangiographic and radionuclide techniques. Circulation **60** 760-6

2. Schnittger I, Fitzgerald P J, Daughters G T, Ingels N B, Kantrowitz
N E, Schwarzkopf A, Mead C W and Popp R L 1982   Limitations of
comparing left ventricular volumes by two-dimensional echocardiography,
myocardial markers and cineangiography. Am.J. Cardiol. **50** 512-19

3. Lapido G O A, Dunn F G, Pringle T H, Bastian B and Lawrie T V D
1980   Serial measurements of left ventricular dimensions by
echocardiography. Br. Heart J. **44** 284-9

4.   Martin M A and Fieller N R J 1979   Echocardiography in
cardiovascular drug assessment. Br. Heart J. **41** 536- 43

5. Shapiro E, Marier D L, St John Sutton M G and Gibson D G 1980
Regional non-uniformity of wall dynamics in the normal left ventricle.
Br. Heart J. **45** 1264-70

6.   Upton M T and Gibson D G 1978   The study of left ventricular function from digitized echocardiograms.   Prog. Cardiovasc. Dis. **20** 359-84

7.   Gibson D G and Brown D J 1975   Measurement of peak rates of left ventricular wall movement in man.   Comparison of echocardiography and angiocardiography. Br. Heart J. **37** 677-83

8.   Traill T A and Gibson D G 1979   Left ventricular relaxation and fillings: study by echocardiography.   In Yu P N and Goodwin J F (eds) Progress in Cardiology, Lea and Febiger, Philadelphia, Vol.8 pp 39-72

9.   Chen W and Gibson D G 1979   Relation of isovolumic relaxation to left ventricular wall movement in man. Br. Heart J. **42** 51-6

10. Mattheos M, Shapiro E, Oldershaw P J Sacchetti R and Gibson D G 1982   Non-invasive assessment of changes in left ventricular relaxation by combined phono-, echo-, and mechanography. Br. Heart J. **47**   253-60

11.   Traill T A, Gibson D G and Brown D J 1978   Study of left ventricular wall thickness and dimension changes using echocardiography. Br. Heart J. **40** 162-9

12.   Gibson D G, Traill T A, Hall R J C and Brown D J 1979 Echocardiographic features of secondary left ventricular hypertrophy. Br. Heart J. **41** 54-9

13.   St John Sutton M G, St John Sutton M, Oldershaw P, Sacchetti R, Paneth M, Lennox S C, Gibson R V and Gibson D G 1981   Valve replacement without cardiac catheterization. N. Engl. J. Med. **305** 1233-8

14.   Gibson D G and Brown D J 1976   Assessment of left ventricular systolic function in man from simultaneous echocardiographic and pressure measurements. Br. Heart J. **38** 8-17

15.   Dawson J R and Sutton G C 1981   Detection of clinically significant coronary artery disease in hypertensive patients. Br. Heart J. **46** 595-602

16.   Gibson D G, Brown D J and Logan-Sinclair R B 1978   Analysis of regional left ventricular wall movement by phased array echocardiography. Br. Heart J. **40** 1334-8

Basic Techniques in Doppler Cardiology

R Skidmore

Department of Medical Physics, Bristol General Hospital, Guinea Street, Bristol

1. Introduction

The noninvasive measurement of blood velocity in peripheral vessels by Doppler ultrasound has become well established over the last twenty years. However, it is only very recently that the investigation of cardiac disorders has attracted the use of Doppler ultrasound as a diagnostic modality. This relatively late demand has been primarily due to the inadequate design of Doppler signal processing instrumentation.

The recent addition of Doppler to 2-D ultrasonic imaging systems and the improvement in Doppler signal processing has stimulated an interest in this field.

It is the purpose of this paper to review the basic currently available technology and illustrate its possible use with some clinical examples.

2. The Doppler Effect

The Doppler effect is the apparent change in observed frequency of a moving source of sound relative to the observer. The classical example often given is the increase in pitch, heard at the station, of a train's whistle as it approaches, and the decrease in pitch as it leaves. The Doppler effect contains information about the train's velocity and direction, providing the pitch of the whistle is already known. This same effect can be used with ultrasound to obtain noninvasive information about the direction and velocity of blood within the body.

3. Doppler Devices

3.1 Continuous Wave (CW)

This technique consists of transmitting a continuous beam of ultrasound at a fixed frequency, usually 2-3 MHz, into the body using a piezoelectric crystal and receiving the resultant backscattered Doppler shifted ultrasound from moving blood on another crystal. The CW velocimeter compares the frequency of the received signal with that of the transmitted signal, the consequent output being an audio signal whose frequency is the Doppler shift frequency for the relative velocity of backscatterers within the ultrasound beam. The Doppler shift frequency, F_d, is related to velocity of the backscattering blood cells by;

$$F_d = \frac{2FV\cos\Theta}{C} \tag{1}$$

where F = transmitter frequency, V = velocity of backscatterers
Θ = the angle between the transmitted sound beam and the direction
of flow, and C = the velocity of the sound in the medium (1540 m/sec).
For absolute velocity measurement angle Θ must be known.

As negative frequencies cannot exist in reality, as would be the case for
relative motion away from the probe, the Doppler velocimeter overcomes
this problem by quadrature demodulation which provides two audio
outputs phase shifted by + or - 90° depending on whether there are +ve
or -ve Doppler shift frequencies present. These two outputs are then
processed by various analog or digital techniques to provide a visual
display of the Doppler shift information.

The disadvantage of CW Doppler is that any motion in the path of the
the beam   produces a Doppler shift. Fig. 1 illustrates how the positive
flow of the mitral valve and the negative flow of the left ventricle are
both recorded when using CW.

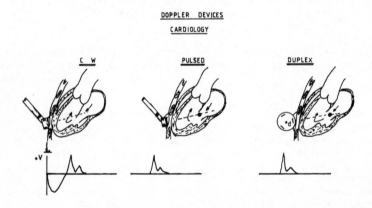

Fig. 1 Doppler devices in use in Cardiology

3.2 Pulsed Doppler

Depth discrimination can be achieved by using a Pulsed Doppler system.
Simply, this consists of a CW device modified so that the transmitting
crystal sends out a burst of ultrasound which is then received on the
same crystal which also acts as a receiver. The output of the receiver
is then sampled at a rate corresponding to the time it takes for the
transmitted pulses to leave the transmitting crystal and return from the
depth of interest.

Although this technique has the advantage of being able to sample

velocities at various depths in the body it suffers from the major
disadvantage of having an upper limit set on the maximum velocity it can
interrogate. So that confusion does not occur, the pulsed Doppler only
sends out a burst of pulses after it has received the information from
the depth of interest, increasing depth requires a longer wait. The time
between bursts or sampling rate is known as the pulse repetition
frequency (PRF). The maximum Doppler shift frequency that can be
measured, Fmax, is given by;

$$\text{Fmax} = \frac{\text{PRF}}{2} \tag{2}$$

A conflict now exists between range and maximum velocity, an increase
in range means a decrease in the maximum measurable velocity. Velocities
that exceed this limit present the user with the inability to assess
magnitude and direction.

Fig. 1 illustrates how the pulsed system with its range gate placed in
the mitral valve orifice does not "see" the velocities within the left
ventricle outflow tract.

3.3 Duplex

This is a combination of real-time 2D ultrasonic imaging and pulsed
Doppler. The advantage of such a system is that the real-time image
can be used to locate the position of the Doppler range gate thus
eliminating the need to guide the Doppler beam by "ear".

Because the imaging head doubles up as the Doppler transducer, (Fig. 1),
there can sometimes be difficulty in obtaining Doppler signals from
the ascending aorta when insonated from the supra-sternal notch due to
the size of the duplex probe.

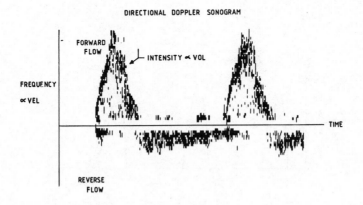

DIRECTIONAL DOPPLER SONOGRAM

Fig. 2 Directional Doppler Sonogram

4. Presentation of Doppler information

4.1 Spectral Analysis

The Doppler signal consists of an audio signal whose frequencies
correspond to the relative velocity of blood cells within the ultrasound
beam. By using an audio spectrum analyser it is possible to display
the distribution of velocities as a function of time, in the form of a
frequency/time plot, commonly known as a sonogram (see Fig 2). The
intensity of the display corresponds to the amount of blood. Most
commercially available Doppler spectrum analysers employ a real-time
FFT hard-wired system, allowing the blood velocity/time distribution
to be observed instantaneously.

4.2 Analogue Processing Systems

Although spectral analyses provide the user with a complete picture
of the Doppler signal, especially in highlighting artifacts such as wall
or valve movement, it is expensive.

Two analogue systems have been developed which extract two important
parameters from the Doppler signal, the instantaneous mean and maximum
frequency. Fig. 3 illustrates the output of an analogue mean and maximum
system when fed with a signal from a pulsed Doppler whose sample volume
has been placed in the ascending aorta. One particular advantage of
using a mean frequency processor in the ascending aorta is that the
area under the curve is directly proportional to the stroke volume,
providing the insonating beam of ultrasound is sufficiently wide enough
to cover the vessel lumen. The maximum frequency follower, however, is
only of use if a spectrum analyser is not available.

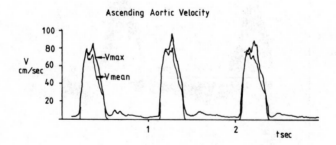

Fig. 3 Analogue maximum and mean velocity traces
from the ascending aorta of a normal subject.

5.   Clinical Applications

Doppler cardiology is still in its infancy where much of the information obtained is used in a qualitative manner. Although quantification is extremely desirable, much work has yet to be done.

The basic qualitative signs the Doppler investigator would look for in diagnosing abnormalities within the heart fall into three areas:-

(i)   Change in waveform shape from the normal

(ii)   Flow direction

(iii)   Turbulent flow patterns and jets.

In order to illustrate some possible uses of Doppler cardiology, three examples have been chosen.

5.1 Mitral Stenosis

Fig. 4 illustrates a 2D image of the aortic valve, mitral valve, left atrium and left ventricle. The enlarged left atrium indicates the possibility of mitral stenosis. The Doppler velocity pattern was obtained using a 2 MHz hand held continuous wave probe. The transducer was aligned along the axis of maximum velocity from the apex of the heart.

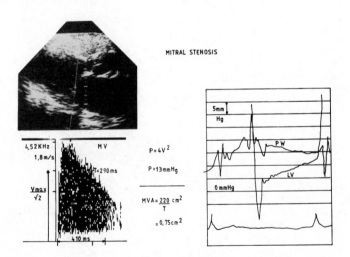

Fig. 4   2D image, Doppler sonogram and pressure
trace - mitral stenosis.

Continuous wave was chosen as the velocity of the stenotic jet was too high for a pulsed system to measure. The velocity pattern consists of a fast rise in early diastole followed by a slow decay.

The Trandheim group (Hatle et al, 1978) have shown that by measuring the absolute peak velocity it is possible to predict, noninvasively, the peak pressure drop using the formula;

$$P = 4v^2$$

where V is the velocity in metre/sec and P is the pressure drop in mmHg. Using this formula in this example, a peak pressure drop of 13 mmHg is predicted which compares well with the catheter peak pressure drop of 15 mmHg illustrated on the right of Fig. 4. Because the pressure drop across the valve will depend on cardiac output, the same group have used another index based on measuring the time, T, taken for the mitral valve velocity to drop to 0.707   ($1/\sqrt{2}$) of its peak velocity. They claim by using this information, it enables them to estimate mitral valve area (MVA) using the formula

$$MVA = \frac{220}{T} \text{ where T is msec.}$$

For this example we see that the mitral valve area is predicted to be 0.75 cm^2.

5.2 Atrial Septal Defect (ASD)

Fig. 5 illustrates pulmonary and aortic average velocity obtained using a hand held pulsed Doppler. By measuring the corresponding area under the curves it may be possible to noninvasively quantify the shunt. The assumption here is that the diameter of pulmonary and aortic arteries are equal.

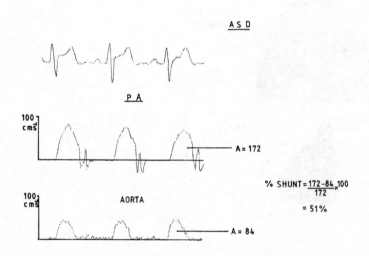

Fig. 5 Pulmonary and aortic average velocity traces - ASD

5.3 Aortic Valve Disease

Fig. 6 illustrates how the sample volume of pulsed Doppler may be guided to sit behind the aortic valve. The Doppler pattern exibits severe disturbed reverse flow during systole, confirming the presence of aortic regurgitation.

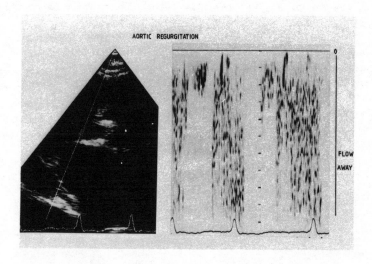

Fig. 6   2D image and Doppler sonogram for sample volume placed behind the aortic valve illustrating aortic regurgitation.

Fig. 7 has been recorded from the ascending aorta in a patient suffering from both aortic stenosis and regurgitation. The shape of the spectrum immediately confirms the diagnosis, the slow disturbed systolic rise and reverse flow in diastole.

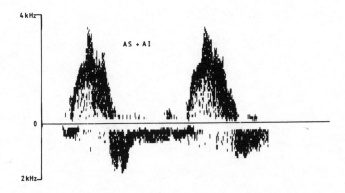

Fig. 7 Doppler sonogram from the ascending aorta - aortic stenosis and regurgitation.

6. Conclusion

No attempt has been made to completely review the whole of Doppler
cardiology, but it is hoped that some of the basics have been outlined,
and that the few examples given may stimulate interest in this rapidly
advancing field.

References

Hatle L, Brabakk A, Tromsdal A, Angelsen B. Noninvasive assessment of
pressure drop in mitral stenosis by Doppler ultrasound. Br Heart J 40:
131, 1978.

Ultrasound Tissue Characterisation of the Heart

S. Leeman

Department of Medical Physics, Hammersmith Hospital and Royal Postgraduate Medical School, London, W12 0HS.

I. Introduction

Ultrasound imaging of the heart at present operates on the pulse-echo principle. A short pulse of ultrasound is generated by a transducer and travels through tissue. On traversing changes in the acoustical properties of the tissue, some of the ultrasound pulse energy is scattered or reflected, and those (back-)scattered waves which are detected by the transducer, now operating as a receiver, are registered as "echoes". On the assumption that a single value (in practice, 1540 ms^{-1}) can be ascribed to the ultrasound propagation velocity in blood and most soft tissues, the distance of a reflecting structure can be estimated from a measurement of the echo return-time. In this way (see "Imaging Techniques with Ultrasound", in this volume) a single line of an image of the region of interest can be obtained. The collection of many such lines constitutes the final image, which can be obtained on a time-scale that may be sufficiently small to effectively freeze the motion of a rapidly moving organ, such as the heart. Thus, by sequentially displaying many such frames, unblurred moving images of cardiac motion can be obtained ("real-time" imaging).

The success of echo cardiographic techniques has depended largely on the ability of ultrasound pulse-echo methods to display relatively accurate cross-sectional cardiac anatomy, and its change throughout the cardiac cycle. Thus, the thickness of the interventricular septum, the presence of an epicardial effusion, the size of a cardiac chamber, or the extent and velocity of movement of a valve leaflet, are all well known examples of the type of information that may be extracted from cardiac B-scan or M-scan "images". The purpose of the ultrasound equipment, and the aim towards which it is designed, is to provide a mapping of detectable echo-generating structures. From this point of view, it is of relatively minor importance to measure whether a particular structure is a strong or weak reflector of ultrasound energy, or even, at a deeper level, to enquire what different processes are operative in generating ultrasound scattering.

In recent years, there has been a growing awareness that, because ultrasound interactions with tissues are complex, the echo from a reflecting or scattering structure contains a great deal of information about the physical composition of that structure, in addition to merely providing an estimate of its distance from the transducer ("range"). Ultrasonic tissue characterization is the attempt to uncover that additional information, and to utilise it to medical advantage.

2. Ultrasound Propagation and Scattering in Human Tissues

An ultrasound pulse traverses a uniformly homogeneous tissue at a definite velocity, which has been demonstrated to depend on tissue type, but which spans the relatively narrow range 1450-1650 ms^{-1} for most soft tissues. In general, the velocity of ultrasound increases with the structural protein content of a tissue, and decreases with its water content. Ultrasound tissue velocities are generally considered to be substantially independent of the frequency content of the propagating pulse, although firm experimental evidence for this is lacking in general. When a pulse passes from one acoustically homogeneous region to another, with differing ultrasound velocities, it is observed to be refracted in accordance with the usual laws of wave motion. Refraction effects are of considerable importance when considering the accuracy of range information, but are of little consequence for most tissue characterisation studies: they are therefore not discussed further here.

In most soft tissues, absorption of ultrasound energy from a passing pulse is very noticeable. "Absorption" refers to the conversion of that energy into heat. Some energy is removed from the forward propagating pulse by being redirected into other directions (e.g. by scattering) and, strictly, the term "attenuation" refers to losses from both absorption and scattering processes. Absorption is difficult to measure accurately and, in most cases, attenuation is the investigated parameter. In general, attenuation in soft tissues drops with increasing water content and rises with increasing structural protein content. In contrast to ultrasound velocity, attenuation, α, in mammalian soft tissues depends on the ultrasound frequency, f, of the propagating wave:

$$\alpha = af^n$$

The constants a and n depend on tissue type, and the index, n, is close to unity in most cases.

Ultrasound pulses are reflected at interfaces between two tissues with different (mean) acoustic propagation parameters. Such reflections are usually interpreted on the basis of a simple physical model, in which only the characteristic acoustic impedance mismatch and the angle of incidence are of importance. Indeed, this is probably the most widely-known description of ultrasound interactions in tissues. In practice, however, this conventional view is woefully inadequate to describe the variety of factors contributing to the reflectivity characteristics of tissue interfaces. Thus, not only do the geometry and orientation of the interface and the impedance mismatch across it determine the reflectivity, but also the absorption mismatch, interface rigidity and microstructure, and possible layering and thickness of the effective boundary region contribute.

An examination of an unmodified 'in vivo' echo sequence will show that, in addition to the relatively isolated, strong and directionally-dependent reflections from large tissue boundaries, there are present also numerous overlapping and relatively weak and directionally-independent echoes originating from within the bulk, rather than boundaries, of tissues. The latter type of echoes are always seen with sensitive equipment, provided that the interrogated tissue is inhomogeneous, and are generally selectively enhanced to constitute the dominant feature of the so-called 'grey scale' image display. Such echoes are interpreted as originating from ultrasound pulse scattering (i.e. redirection into directions other than

the incident) from small acoustic inhomogeneities within tissue. Theoretical considerations predict that these inhomogeneities are spatial or
temporal fluctuations in the local density, elasticity and/or absorption of
the tissue. (An equivalent description is to consider ultrasound scattering as being generated by inhomogeneities in acoustic impedance, velocity
and absorption.) Ultrasound scattering from human tissues is poorly
investigated at present, but it is almost certainly frequency dependent -
as the changes in character of ultrasound grey-scale images attest, when
different imaging frequencies are employed.

Tissue properties which modify the propagation and scattering of ultrasound
pulses are known to be dependent on tissue micro- and molecular structure,
as well as composition, and most have been demonstrated to be dependent on
tissue pathology. Ultrasound echoes from human tissues thus convey information at a level that is not easily perceived in conventional images. A
major problem is, unfortunately, the practicable extraction and measurement
of that information in routine applications.

3. Information Extraction from Ultrasound Signals

There are three ways in which tissue information is extracted from ultrasound signals from human tissues.

i) B-, M-, and A-mode "imaging" map the location, but not the type, of
scattering structures. The aim here is primarily to show detail for visual
assessment, and the raw echoes detected from tissues are extensively processed towards that end. Although grey-scale images present the illusion
of scatterer identification, the brightness of the image is only very
crudely indicative of scatterer strength, and conveys little information
about scatterer type (e.g. density or compressibility variation?). Indeed,
some processing options will enhance images for improved visual acceptance
at the cost of losing fundamental physical information about the tissue:
thus the use of time-gain-compensation enables a larger tissue region to be
satisfactorily imaged, but corrupts the assessment of ultrasound attenuation from the image itself.

ii) Quantitative imaging attempts to map the distribution and strength of a
single ultrasound/tissue interaction parameter, in a truly quantitative
way. "In vivo" impedance, ultrasound velocity, and attenuation maps have
been obtained with research equipment, but specialised scanning, measurement, and computational techniques are necessitated. The methods have
little in common with conventional ultrasound imaging and, inevitably,
recourse to computers must be made in order to generate the final image.
The applicability of quantitative imaging is at present limited to only a
few sites in the body, and only impedance mapping (which can be derived
from back-scattered echo sequences alone) appears to be ultimately applicable to the heart. Doppler imaging may be regarded as a special case of
quantitative imaging, and can produce a map of blood velocity within the
body. However, its use to map intra-cardiac blood velocities would not be
truly quantitative with the commercial scanning equipment presently available.

iii) Tissue characterisation seeks to uncover quantitative and typical
characteristics of the echo sequence which measure the spatial and/or
temporal variation of any tissue property, or mixture of such properties.
It is clear that any such derived characteristic must be intrinsic to the
tissue itself (and not be unduly influenced by scanner properties), and

must be related to tissue pathology or physiological state. Ultrasound is
a particularly convenient modality for tissue characterisation since, not
only do ultrasound echoes carry some information that is not readily measured by other radiations, but also, ultrasound scanning is safe, cheap and
non-traumatic, being widely used and acceptable to both doctors and
patients alike. Moreover, ultrasound scanners can provide high quality
real-time images, in which the tissue region to be investigated can be
rapidly and relatively clearly pin-pointed in most cases. As will be seen
below, tissue characterisation involves the processing of ultrasound echoes,
and the availability of commercial conventional ultrasound scanners with
digital processing and imaging facilities ensures the possibility that
successful characterisation routines will probably be implemented within
the context of routine ultrasound scanning, at very little extra cost. The
aim of tissue characterisation is not necessarily to enhance diagnostic
effectiveness: it has a clear role, in certain situations, in the clinical
management of patients, particularly in monitoring early response to drugs
or surgical manoeuvres. Moreover, tissue characterisation has a clear role
in assessing the severity, or extent, of an already diagnosed condition.

4. General Tissue Characterisation Methods and Problems

Tissue characterisation encompasses a wide variety of techniques which
fall into one of three categories: parameter estimation, structure characterisation, and dynamic tissue characterisation.

Parameter estimation is the quantitative measurement of tissue acoustical
properties; in general, mean values over a region of interest are sought.
Properties of interest include characteristic impedance, ultrasound
velocity, attenuation, and back-scattering strength. In some methods, it
is not the absolute value of the parameter which is measured, but rather
its behaviour with respect to some variable, such as direction (angle) or
frequency. Also in this class are the "echo structure" analyses, which
extract information about changes in mean parameter values across a major
tissue boundary from an analysis of the amplitude and shape of the isolated
echo generated there.

Structure characterisation attempts to assign some index or "signature"
which characterises the spatial distribution of small-scale scattering
structures or their strengths. In practice, such investigations are
carried out on either images or A-scan lines. Thus, the "texture" of the
grey-scale image of a region may be quantified, or the statistics of the
echo amplitudes in that region may be evaluated. The same computations
may be carried out with A-scan lines rather than image regions.

Dynamic tissue characterisation is particularly appropriate in cardiac
studies and characterises the time behaviour (throughout the cardiac cycle,
say) of easily measured echo or tissue signatures. The hope of the dynamic
approach is that the quantitation of time changes within tissue is diagnostically significant and less sensitive to artefact than the quantitation
of the tissue parameters, or structural signatures, themselves.

The problems besetting the successful implementation of tissue characterisation are legion and are not, indeed, all fully understood. Since most
analyses are conducted with pulse-echo data, it is clear that tissues overlying the region of interest may considerably distort or hide the information encoded in the echoes. Echo detection and signal processing procedures implemented in the ultrasound scanner may grossly affect displayed

echo characteristics. The choice of transducer and machine settings may
also distort echo information. Some compensation for these effects should
be made, but this is rarely done in most tissue characterisation techniques.
The anisotropy of some organs and tissues makes it difficult to accumulate
consistent data sets from a large number of patients, unless internal
tissue landmarks can be recognised, and the tissues interrogated from a
variety of directions. Tissue movement compromises the ability to obtain
a sufficiently large data set from a pre-selected region of interest only.
In practice, some of these difficulties are confronted by relating the
measured properties of the region of interest to those of "standard"
normal tissues, as monitored within the same patient.

5.   Cardiac Tissue Characterisation

The heart appears to be a good candidate for tissue characterisation investigations. Thus, some forms of myocardial hypertrophy might be expected to
result in tissue density or structural changes, myocardial contractility
changes might result in modified tissue elasticity (compressibility), and
ischaemia and necrosis might modify both tissue absorption and elasticity.
Changes in these tissue properties all influence ultrasound echoes and are,
in principle, amenable to tissue characterisation investigations. Certain
cardiomyopathies are associated with abnormal protein or fluid accumulations,
or with disorganisation of the myofibrils - all amenable to tissue characterisation. Calcification of valve leaflets presents another obvious and
fertile area for investigation.

It is, of course, easy to hint at the potential of a technique, but it is
another matter to demonstrate its feasibility more directly. In fact, there
is available laboratory evidence to suggest that cardiac tissue characterisation is not an empty hope. It has been found that the frequency spectrum
of echoes from muscle tissue is modified after vascular occlusion, that the
frequency dependence of ultrasound attenuation in canine myocardium is correlated with biochemical indices of myocardial infarction, and that both
ultrasound attenuation and back-scattered echo strength are modified by
coronary occlusion of rabbit and canine hearts. In these last experiments,
the attenuation and back-scattering strength were significantly enhanced in
the infarcted area compared with normal, unaffected myocardium, and the
observed changes appear to follow   collagen concentration changes in the
affected tissues. There is also some evidence that the angular dependence
of the back-scattered echo strength from a small region may depend on the
local structural arrangement of the myofibrils. While the available
evidence is certainly not overwhelming in its abundance, and is based on
studies with animal tissues, it is probably quite fair to suggest that
(human) cardiac tissue characterisation has a good chance of success, providing that sufficiently sensitive measurement and processing methods can
be devised for 'in vivo' applications.

There are also isolated, somewhat anecdotal, reports in the literature of
observations made during routine clinical scanning sessions which lend further credence to some of the results referred to above. It is generally
known that echo amplitudes are influenced by mitral valve calcification,
and there is at least one report that calcification may be distinguished
from fibrosis on this basis. It has been observed that the "texture", or
pattern of echoes, of the grey-scale appearance of a tumour such as a
myxoma is somewhat different to that of a sarcoma. It has also been noted
(indeed, by more than one investigator!) that the B-scan texture of the
abnormal interventricular septum is modified by disease, particularly in

cases of amyloidosis and idiopathic hypertrophic subaortic stenosis (IHSS). The observed unusual "ground glass" texture has been attributed to fibrosis and fibre disorientation. It has also been reported, in more than one study, that endocardial plaque may be detected by the intense echoes generated. Few of these observations are backed by firm statistical evidence, but it should be emphasised that they have been made with commercial real-time imaging equipment in which optimal grey-scale display must have been low on the list of design priorities.

6. Cardiac Tissue Characterisation: Some Problems

At present, it is unlikely that success with cardiac tissue characterisation can be achieved without the use of specially modified equipment, in order to extract and analyse echo signals which have not been subjected to the gross distortions necessitated in commercial M- and B-scan equipment. Even given that such technical problems are resolved, there are a number of difficulties associated with the heart itself which demand a more careful design of a tissue characterisation investigation than is required for most other organs in the body. These are briefly reviewed here.

i) Motion: the heart, by its very nature, is constantly in rapid motion. This makes it difficult (and with standard methods, impossible) to track a particular tissue segment to ensure that echoes from that region only are being analysed. The difficulty may be overcome to some extent, in most patients, by simultaneously monitoring the ECG, for example, and ensuring that echoes acquired only during a particular phase of the cardiac cycle are analysed. Such a procedure clearly simplifies the comparison of results between different patients, observers, and even from the same patient, if the time course of some condition is being investigated.

ii) Cycling: even if a specified segment of cardiac tissue could be tracked throughout the cardiac cycle, it is highly unlikely (as experiments with canine hearts confirm) that its measurable acoustic properties and tissue signatures would remain constant throughout the contraction and relaxation phases of the muscle. Here again, utilising the ECG as a "clock" in order to analyse data from only known phases of the cardiac cycle would be advantageous. A direct consequence of this approach, first suggested by the author, is to compare results throughout the cardiac cycle in order to follow the changes in measured properties. Significance is then attached also to the time variation of the tissue characterisation indices, rather than only to their absolute value at a particular cardiac phase. Necrotic or ischaemic regions would be expected to show considerably less time variation than normal regions. Unfortunately it is very difficult, in such a dynamic tissue characterisation approach, to distinguish between the significant cycling and the less-important motion effects. In practice, it is sometimes more convenient to compare results at two phases only (say end-diastole and end-systole) rather than mapping the full-time course throughout the cardiac cycle.

Another approach to handling motion and cycling effects is to devise a technique which measures time-averaged quantities. In some cases, this should simplify the design of equipment and will obviate the need for internal clocks such as the ECG, but it is felt that such a simple-minded technique has little to commend it.

iii) Anisotropy: 'in vitro' (animal) studies have established that cardiac tissue acoustical properties, such as attenuation, are markedly anisotropic.

This unfortunate difficulty may be partially overcome by ensuring that scanning planes and data acquisition directions are accurately and repeatedly obtainable. This is not beyond the competence of a skilled echocardiographer. The measurement of anisotropy, or its absence, may in itself provide a tissue characterisation index, but this has not been attempted in practice.

iv) Acoustic window: the human heart may be (non-invasively) ultrasonically viewed 'in vivo' only through a limited number of relatively small acoustic windows. This severely restricts the full range of information that can be acquired for tissue characterisation and may well exclude some cardiac regions from such investigations. Certain signatures, such as those based on anisotropy assessment and angle dependence of back-scattering strength, may be rendered impotent by acoustic window limitations.

v) Cardiac size: some tissue characterisation methods, which are of potential value in cardiac studies (such as attenuation estimation from back-scattered echoes), require fairly long tissue segments for implementation. Such techniques, as developed for relatively large organs such as the liver, need considerable refinement before they can be implemented on the short data sets obtainable from the myocardium.

It should be appreciated that many of the above problems compromise not only successful implementation of tissue characterisation techniques but, indeed, may be adduced as diluting the value of some conventional echocardiographic studies. The latter have, none-the-less, enjoyed phenomenal advances in recent years. The rapid and pragmatic progress of echocardiography may therefore be interpreted as intimating that cardiac tissue characterisation will not be unduly impeded by these difficulties.

7. Cardiac Tissue Characterisation: Present Methods

It is surprising that so few groups are actively engaged on tissue characterisation studies of patients presenting for echocardiographic investigation. To some extent this may result from a lack of awareness, amongst echocardiographers, of the full range of information latent in the grey-scale image, coupled with the general view that dimensions, velocities, timing of events, and spatial relationships are the most significant features to be probed with ultrasound methods.

It has long been appreciated that the measurement of certain features of an M-scan trace may aid in the diagnosis of certain conditions or in assessing their severity (e.g. measurement of diastolic closure rate). Such investigations may be regarded as incipient tissue characterisation techniques. Chu and Raeside (1978) have extended this approach into a "true" tissue characterisation technique. They have used pattern recognition methods, applied to the whole pattern of motion of the anterior mitral valve cusp, in order to differentiate mitral stenosis from normals. Lewis and Leeman have improved on this by devising a technique based on the correlation analysis of the pattern of motion of both the anterior and posterior leaflets (unpublished work, but see Lewis, 1981). They have found that their method, when applied to mitral stenosis, is somewhat better than existing diagnostic indices such as diastolic closure rate and amplitude of leaflet excursion in distinguishing the diseased from the normal valve. There is also some suggestion that the method can provide an index of degree of stenosis, even in mixed mitral valve disease. As interest in the quantitative evaluation of (digitised) M-scan traces grows, it may be expected that "characterisation of motion" studies will increase apace.

There do not appear to be any systematic quantitative investigations based on the quantitative analysis of isolated echoes as generated from a blood/myocardium interface, or from valve leaflets. It is felt that such studies would be of great value in certain valvular diseases and perhaps in myocardial investigations: perhaps the near future will see this unhappy state of affairs remedied.

Certain doppler investigations are readily classed as tissue characterisation studies but these are not discussed here (see "Basic Techniques in Doppler Cardiology", in this volume).

Two groups have investigated the pattern of echoes from within the myocardium in order to arrive at a tissue characterisation index. Joynt et al (1980) have analysed the distribution of echo amplitudes obtained from normal human subjects and myocardial infarction cases. Although the number of subjects was very small, these authors felt that the analysis provided a differentiation between normal and affected myocardium. Another approach by these authors involves the characterisation of the spectra of the returned echoes by forming the autocorrelation of the power spectra of the back-scattered sequence; they found clear differences between end-diastolic and end-systolic patterns in both normals and subjects with IHSS (HOCM). Leeman et al (1980) have analysed the back-scattered echo sequence from the interventricular septum of both normals and HOCM cases. They have found that the autocorrelation of the returned echo envelope (A-scan) changes markedly between the end-diastolic and end-systolic phases in both (small) sets of patients, and that such an autocorrelation analysis provides a discrimination between normal and diseased states.

8. Cardiac Tissue Characterisation: The Future?

There is some laboratory evidence, based on 'in vitro' and 'in vivo' animal studies, to suggest that cardiac tissue characterisation is feasible. It is surprising and disappointing that this, and the general interest in tissue characterisation, have not generated more extensive and systematic studies with human patients. With some modification to existing equipment, it is possible to acquire data for tissue characterisation during routine echocardiographic examinations without any inconvenience to the patient. It is inconceivable that cardiac tissue characterisation will not develop rather more rapidly now than in the past. The widespread use of real-time grey-scale scanners and colour-coded images, and the availability of powerful, low-cost micro-computers, will almost certainly kindle enthusiasm amongst cardiologists and scientists alike. Tissue characterisation has the potential to become one of the standard and routine techniques of echocardiography in the not too distant future.

9. References

Chu W K and Raeside D E 1978 Phys. Med. Biol. 23(1) 100.
Joynt L, Martin R and Macovski A 1980 Acoustical Imaging 8 ed A Metherell (New York: Plenum) pp527-38.
Leeman S, Gehrke J, Hutchins L and Sutton P 1980 Ultrasonic Tissue Characterisation ed J M Thijssen (Brussels: Stafleu) pp117-23.
Lewis L M 1981 Brit. J. Radiol. 54 541.

A complete, if somewhat concise and techhical, review of tissue characterisation methods is presented in:

Leeman S and Jones J P 1982 Proc. 1st IEEE Computer Society Int. Symp. on
   Medical Imaging and Image Interpretation (IEEE Cat. No. 82CH1804-4; Comp.
   Soc. Order No. 438) (Silver Spring: IEEE Computer Society Press) pp179-84.

Another, less critical, review of tissue characterisation methods is:

Linzer M and Norton S J 1982 Ann. Rev. Biophys. Bioeng. 11 303.

Radionuclides in Cardiology: An Overview

A.T. Elliott

West of Scotland Health Boards, Dept. of Clinical Physics & Bioengineering,
Western Infirmary, Glasgow G11 6NT.

Abstract. Nuclear cardiology is now an integral part of the workup of
patients with a wide range of cardiac disorders. The various
examinations involve the administration of a radioactive material whose
passage through, or distribution within, the heart is monitored by
means of a scintillation probe or (more usually) a gamma camera. There
are three major investigations in current use - the radionuclide
angiocardiogram, infarct imaging and myocardial perfusion imaging. A
brief description of each technique is given, along with a discussion
of the equipment required and an overview of their clinical
application.

1. Introduction

Nuclear cardiology is concerned with the assessment of cardiac function
rather than anatomy and is one of the largest and fastest growing areas of
nuclear medicine. It had its beginnings with the work of Prinzmetal and
his colleagues (1948), who used a Geiger counter positioned over the
precordium to generate a graph recording the passage of a bolus of
sodium-24 through the right and left sides of the heart. The temporal
resolution of their system was two data points per second and the
statistics associated with their data were poor. Today's radionuclide
angiocardiogram consists of cardiac images recorded at framing rates of up
to 100 per second and counting rates nearing 500000 per second; ejection
fraction, ventricular filling and emptying rates and ventricular wall
motion patterns are some of the parameters which may be obtained.
Investigations have been developed for the diagnosis of myocardial
infarction and to study myocardial perfusion and metabolism: the
relatively recent advent of positron imaging devices has led to
particularly exciting developments in the latter area.

2. Technical considerations

2.1 Radiopharmaceuticals

The radiopharmaceuticals most commonly employed for each of the above
tests are shown in Table 1. With the exception of thalium -201, they emit
gamma radiation, this being the type of radiation which is least absorbed
in the body: at 140keV, the photon energy of technetium-99m, the half
value thickness in tissue is about 45mm. In the case of thallium-201, it
is the 79keV X-ray photon which is detected. At this energy, many photons
are absorbed within the patient, particularly those from the posterior

surfaces of the heart. Technetium-99m is the radionuclide incorporated into most radiopharmaceuticals because of its ready availability from a molybdenum/technetium generator. Its chemistry is complex, however, due to its high valency state. Monovaler iodine is chemically easier to incorporate into a pharmaceutical but the previously available isotope, iodine-131, has an 8-day half-life and emits beta, in addition to gamma, radiation; both factors lead to a high patient radiation dose. Within the past few years, iodine-123 has become available, with markedly superior dosimetric properties. Among the more successful radiopharmaceuticals labelled with this radioisotope are the fatty acids, hexa- and hepta-decenoic acid, which have been brought into routine clinical use (Freundlieb et al.,1980) for myocardial perfusion/metabolism studies. Much effort is being devoted to agents which might replace thallium-201, which has poor imaging and dosimetry properties, and some other iodine-123 compounds still at the development stage show promise, such as the guanethidine analogue meta- iodobenzyl guanidine (Wieland et al., 1981: Kline et al., 1981). Technetium-99m complexes such as DMPE (Deutsch et al., 1982) are under investigation also.

Radiopharmaceuticals used for positron imaging usually incorporate ^{11}C, ^{13}N, ^{15}O, ^{18}F or ^{68}Ga. Blood pool imaging has been carried out with carbon monoxide incorporating ^{11}C (Phelps et al., 1976) and with ^{68}Ga-labelled red cells (Welch et al., 1977). Myocardial metabolism has been investigated using ^{18}F 2-deoxyglucose (Phelps et al., 1978; Ratib et al., 1982), ^{11}C palmitate (Weiss et al., 1977) and $^{13}N/^{11}C$-labelled amino acids (Henze et al., 1982).

2.2 Detector systems

Gamma radiation is detected by means of scintillation devices, the scintillator in common use for in vivo measurements being thallium-activated sodium iodide (NaI(Tl)). In a probe device, a NaI(Tl) crystal up to 75mm diameter and 75mm deep is viewed by a single photomultiplier, the field of view being defined by a large bore collimator. Such detectors do not yield an image, only an activity-time curve, and were used to obtain the first routine nuclear angiocardiograms (Conn, 1962; Donato, Guintini and Lewis, 1962).

In the conventional design of gamma camera (Anger, 1958) a large NaI(Tl) crystal, 13mm thick and up to 550m diameter, is viewed by an array of photomultiplier tubes arranged in concentric hexagonal rings around a central tube. The geometrical field of view is limited by a multi-hole collimator placed over the front of the crystal: a gamma photon passing through the collimator interacts to produce a light flash in the crystal. The photomultiplier signals are dependent on their position relative to the light flash and can be processed to give the co-ordinates, relative to arbitrary X and Y axes, of the event. Further, by summing the photo-multiplier output signals, an "energy" signal is obtained which can be sub-mitted to pulse-height analysis to exclude events due to scattered photons. Those events accepted by the energy analysis are recorded as a dot on an oscilloscope screen at a location determined by the X and Y co-ordinates. The image is obtained by making a time exposure photograph of the oscillo-scope and is comprised typically of 500,000 dots. Alternatively, the X and Y co-ordinates are fed to a computer via individual analogue-to-digital converters and the image stored in matrix form. The size of matrix varies according to the investigation: for a static study, 128×128 or 256×256 element arrays would be used while for dynamics, 32×32 or 64×64 arrays suffice.

Table 1 Radiopharmaceuticals used in nuclear cardiology

Investigation	Radiopharmaceutical
Acute infarct imaging	Tc-99m pyrophosphate
Myocardial perfusion imaging	
(a) invasive	Kr-81m, Xe-133
	Tc-99m microspheres
(b) non-invasive	Tl-201
	I-123 fatty acids
	positron radiopharmaceuticals
Nuclear angiocardiography	
(a) gated equilibrium	Tc-99m albumin
	Tc-99m red blood cells
(b) first pass	Tc-99m pertechnetate
	Tc-99m red blood cells
	Au-195m

Table 2 Role of the pyrophosphate scan

1. Infarct diagnosis
   (a) equivocal/unreliable enzymes
   (b) ECG conduction defects
   (c) perioperative infarction
   (d) right ventricular infarction

2. Myocardial contusion

3. Infarct sizing (ECAT)

4. Prognosis

5. Pericarditis

Table 3 Role of the myocardial perfusion scan

1. Detection and evaluation of coronary artery disease

2. Identification of false-positive exercise ECG

3. Assessment of significance of identified coronary stenoses

4. Assessment pre- and post-CABG: follow-up

5. Prognosis

6. Investigation of myocardial metabolism

7. Infarct sizing (ECAT)

8. Sarcoidosis

An alternative design is that of the multicrystal gamma camera
(Bender and Blau, 1962) which utilises a matrix of small independent
NaI(Tl) crystals. Light from each crystal is fed through an extremely
complex light guide system to two photomultipliers, there being a photomultiplier for each row and each column of the matrix: event location is
determined by coincidence analysis of the row and column signals. Counts
are stored initially in a CMOS buffer memory prior to transfer into the
integral computer. In this system, only digital images are available.

Recently, the probe has re-appeared, now coupled to a microcomputer
(Wagner et al., 1976). This appears to be useful in the continuous
assessment of global ventricular function in response to drugs etc
(Berger et al., 1981).

Emission tomography using conventional "single photon" radiopharmaceuticals, which dates from the work of Kuhl and Edwards in 1963,
has become widely practised only very recently with the advent of
rotating camera systems (Jaszczak et al., 1977) and the multiple pinhole
collimator (Vogel et al., 1979. The latter technique is now
generally accepted to show no substantial advantage over planar imaging
(see section 4 below). Early rotating camera systems were hampered by
technical problems and, while many of these have been overcome, no
convincing data have been presented to demonstrate added advantages of
this technique.   In particular, the goal of absolute quantification
of radiopharmaceutical uptake has not been attained.

Positron tomography requires the detection of 511keV annihilation photon
pairs in opposed detector pairs. Commercial systems employ dual
rotating cameras (Muehllehner, Buchin and Dubek, 1976) or an hexagonal
array of detectors (Hoffman et al., 1976). Such systems are themselves
extremely expensive and, as yet, require the provision of an on-site
cyclotron. They thus appear to be restricted to research applications in
a few major centres.

3. Myocardial infarct imaging

Acute infarct imaging gained widespread acceptance during the early 1970's
with the introduction of ^{99m}Tc-labelled complexes, particularly the
phosphates (Bonte et al., 1974). These were found to accumulate in
infarcted myocardium, achieving maximal concentration in damaged tissues
some 24-48 hours post infarction. Wackers et al., (1976) used
thallium-201 to produce a negative image of infarcted areas very soon
(less than 6 hours) after the acute event, but this radiopharmaceutical
cannot distinguish between old and new infarcts and fails to visualise at
least one-third of subendocardial lesions (Pitt and Strauss, 1976). A
comparative study by Grossman et al., (1977) suggested that
imidodiphosphonate might permit earlier imaging than other phosphates, a
suggestion confirmed by Ell et al., (1978), but the radiopharmaceutical of
choice has remained ^{99m}Tc-pyrophosphate (PYP) (Olson et al., 1979;
Holman et al., 1980). Injection should be made directly into a vein and
not through tubing since PYP has a tendency to adhere to plastic. Images
should be obtained one hour post injection in at least four projections
(AP, LAO 30, LAO 55 and LLAT) to obtain maximum information: repeat images
may be necessary 2 or 3 hours post injection if the blood clearance is
delayed as in patients with poor renal function. Interpretation of the
images is usually carried out following the method of Willerson et al.
(1975) in which absence of cardiac uptake or diffuse uptake of low

intensity are regarded as negative, grades 0 and 1 respectively, (the latter may be found in the angina patient). Three positive grades, 2-4, are defined as focal areas of increased uptake whose intensities are less than, equal to or greater than that of uptake in the sternum. The scan is most reliable in the period 24 hours - 7 days following the acute event.

Recent developments in ECG mapping and, more particularly, in enzyme assays such as the MB-CK (eg Roberts, Sobel and Parker, 1978; Shell et al., 1979) have rendered infarct imaging largely obsolete in the diagnostic realm with the exception of the situations listed under item 1 of table 2. In conjunction with ECAT techniques, the pyrophosphate scan has been used in an attempt to quantify infarct size (Keyes et al., 1978; Stokeley et al., 1979) but this is of dubious validity. Similarly, the prognostic significance of the scan has been investigated but reduces to the not surprising conclusion that those patients suffering large infarcts have a poor prognosis.

An as yet unproven use for the pyrophosphate scan lies in the detection of endocarditis (Wong et al., 1982). Experience to date in several centres yields conflicting reports: in the author's institution, false negative results have been obtained consistently.

4. Perfusion imaging

Early attempts at myocardial perfusion imaging utilised rubidium-86 (Carr et al., 1962), caesium-131(Carr et al., 1964) and potassium-43 (Hurley et al., 1971). The "gold standard" technique remains the microsphere technique (eg Ritchie et al., 1976) but this is commonly employed now only in the experimental animal as a reference against which other methods are validated. Myocardial capillary blood flow rates can be measured by the injection of an inert gas such as xenon-133 (Holman et al., 1974) or krypton-81m (Selwyn et al., 1980) but these must be administered through a catheter, usually at the time of a contrast angiogram. The most commonly used agent today is thallium-201, introduced by Lebowitz and his colleagues (1973).

Thallium is a potassium analog and acts as a substitute in the sodium-potassium-ATPase system. Ischaemic areas therefore appear as defects or "cold spots" and several investigators (eg Mueller et al., 1976; Nielson et al., 1979) have shown that initial defects in thallium scans are produced predominantly by reduction in blood flow, alterations in extraction fraction playing a secondary role. Thallium-201 is imaged using the 69-83keV X-rays consequent on its decay to mercury (gamma cameras fitted with multiple energy analysers may use the 167 and 135keV γ-rays also) and must be carried out within an interval after production specified by the manufacturer. The production process produces small quantities of Tl-200 (half-life 26 hrs) and Tl-202 (half-life 288 hrs): a delay in use permits decay of the Tl-200 relative to the Tl-201 (half-life 73.5 hours) but, if the delay is too long, the percentage of Tl-202 increases to an unacceptable level. Some investigators (eg Royal, Brown and Claunch, 1979) propound the use of gamma cameras with 6mm thick crystals on the grounds that improved resolution is obtained.

Pohost et al., (1977) demonstrated that the distribution of thallium in the myocardium does not remain static but could change as a function of time following administration during exercise: imaging in patients without infarction but suffering exercise-induced ischaemia demonstrated defects

immediately post-exercise which had "disappeared" when imaging was
repeated four hours later. Defects due to infarction do not resolve.
Beller and Pohost (1977) found that the redistribution phenomenon was due
to a continuous exchange with thallium circulating in the blood pool,
giving rise to washout from normal tissue and accumulation into previously
underperfused areas. It is routine to inject thallium at maximal exercise,
using a graded treadmill or bicycle ergometer protocol, and to continue
the exercise for approximately a minute post-injection to maximise cardiac
blood flow: splanchnic uptake can be minimised by fasting the patient for
at least 6 hours before the test. Initial imaging should begin
immediately after termination of exercise and should comprise AP, LAO 30,
LAO 60 and LLAT views: because of the poor image statistics, the data are
usually recorded by a computer for subsequent processing. Imaging is
repeated four hours after injection, the patient being requested not to
exercise and to eat sparingly in the interval.

Many attempts at processing have been made to improve the diagnostic
accuracy of thallium investigations ranging from image enhancement with
quantification of zonal uptake (Bodenheimer et al.,1978) and image
normalisation with quantification (Murray et al., 1979) to statistical
image analysis (Faris et al., 1982). Seven pinhole tomography has been
widely used also (eg Vogel, et al 1979; Berman et al., 1980).
No single processing method for planar imaging has gained widespread
acceptance: the only point of agreement is that some form of processing
is an improvement on qualitative inspection of the analogue images, as
would be expected from past quality data. There is no agreement either
as to whether tomographic imaging is advantageous - Francisco et al.
(1982) felt it improved predictive accuracy while Faris et al. (1982)
found quantitave planar imaging superior. A somewhat more promising
application of mathematics to thallium imaging is the application of
Bayesian analysis (Hamilton et al., 1978).

Nevertheless, the thallium scan is probably the most commonly performed
nuclear cardiology investigation. It is used for all the purposes shown
in table 3 with the exception of item 6, for which other agents, such as
the radioiodinated fatty acids, are being developed. Absolute measures of
metabolism can be carried out with positron emitting agents and will be
described later (Selwyn, these Proceedings).

Long chain fatty acids are an important energy source for the myocardium
and are efficiently extracted from the blood. Their potential use as a
direct probe of B-oxidation has led to much research effort, although Otto
et al. (1981) have shown that for chain lengths greater than 15, the
cellular fate of fatty acids is predominantly triglyceride storage. Using
heptadecenoic acid, coupled with a correction for activity not specifically bound, Freundlieb et al. (1980) and Abdullah et al. (1981) showed that
significant differences in washout rate occur in patients with coronary
artery disease. Further work remains to elucidate the precise mechanisms
being investigated, but the technique shows promise.

5. Nuclear angiocardiography

This investigation has come to occupy a major role in cardiology as both a
routine clinical and a research tool as can be seen from tables 4 and 5.
Both of the currently-used techniques, first-pass and multiple-gated
imaging, have proven reliable for the non-invasive assessment of left
ventricular ejection fraction and wall motion (eg Dymond et al., 1982;

Table 4   Role of resting nuclear angiogram

1. Evaluation of cardiomegaly

2. Detection of LV aneurysms (true and false)

3. Differentiation of aneurysms from diffuse hypokinesis

4. Assessment of extent of myocardial infarction

5. Evaluation of cardiac function in patients on cytotoxic chemotherapy

6. LV function measurements when contrast angiography impracticable

7. Evaluation of RV function

8. Baseline information for longitudinal follow-up

Table 5   Role of the exercise nuclear angiogram

1. Evaluation of patients with chest pain

2. Physiological assessment of dubious coronary stenoses

3. Efficacy of coronary artery surgery, thrombolysis or PTCA

4. Physiological assessment of non-coronary syndromes (LBBB,
   cardiomyopathies etc)

5. Investigation of exercise response to drug therapy

6. Pre-discharge prognostic evaluation of acute MI

7. RV functional reserve in patients with lung disease

8. Longitudinal follow-up

9. Screening of "high-risk" populations

Pfisterer et al., 1979).

In a first-pass study, data are collected at a framing rate of up to 100 images per second for some 30-50 seconds starting simultaneously with the injection of a bolus of radioactivity (eg Marshall et al., 1977). The multiple-gated method (eg Green et al., 1975) requires the use of a non-diffusible radiopharmaceutical, usually the patient's own red blood cells labelled by in vitro (Smith and Richards, 1976) or in vivo (Pavel, Zimmer and Patterson, 1977) techniques, the latter gaining widespread acceptance. In addition to the image data, the patient's ECG is fed to the computer, which is programmed to store the data from successive portions of the cardiac cycle into separate images, storage being reset to the initial image of the sequence each time the QRS complex is identified: provision must be made to reject abnormal cardiac cycles. In both techniques, a study may be performed with the patient at rest or when the heart is subject to stress, usually exercise-induced. An "exercise study" implies a minimum of two measurements, one at exercise and one at rest.

The main disadvantage of the multiple-gated technique is that all chambers of the heart contain radioactive blood simultaneously. This limits the possible image projections to those in which the chamber of interest can be isolated spatially from the remainder of the heart. For the left ventricle, the LAO projection is used primarily: in the RAO projection, the right ventricle masks the inferior wall of the left ventricle. The first-pass method circumvents this problem since separation of the chambers is achieved on a temporal basis: biplane studies, with consequent higher specificity and accuracy (Dymond et al., 1979) are therefore possible.

When carrying out exercise tests by the multiple-gated method, care must be taken to ensure that an adequate number of frames per cardiac cycle is achieved, since the length of the cardiac cycle will vary throughout the text.

The first-pass technique, however is not without drawbacks, the first being that multiple studies require multiple injections of radio-pharmaceutical which increases the radiation dose to the the patient. The multiple-g ated technique allows many studies to be carried out following a single administration of radiopharmaceutical. Secondly, sequential first-pass studies are carried out against a residual radioactive back-ground from preceeding studies, for which a correction must be made. For the correction to be valid, the distribution and amount of background activity must remain constant throughout the subsequent study, which places a constraint on the interval between studies when using technetium. The use of gold-195 m (Elliott et al., 1982) will largely circumvent both of these disadvantages.

When carrying out exercise tests by the multiple-gated method, care must be taken to ensure that an adequate number of frames per cardiac cycle is achieved, since the length of the cardiac cycle will vary throughout the test.

Several technical factors are important in first-pass studies, particularly the integrity of the bolus injection. Dymond et al.,(1982) have shown that bolus volumes greater than 0.5 ml, giving rise to a temporal FWHM of more than a second on passage through the SVC, may lead to unreliable results.

The speed and volume of the saline flush are important also - we have found 8-10 ml per second and 20 mls to be suitable values. Some investigators synchronise injection with the patient's ECG to ensure arrival in the right atrium at the optimum point in the cardiac cycle.

Since data are obtained from the rapid passage (5-8 cycles) of the activity through the left ventricle, first-pass studies may prove difficult in patients with significant arrythmias. In such cases, it may be advantageous to carry out the first-pass study using a non-diffusible radiopharmaceutical so that a subsequent multiple-gated investigation can be undertaken should the initial study prove unsatisfactory.

Of all the parameters which can be measured, those of proven clinical value are the ejection fraction and, more importantly, wall motion images. It is crucial that individual investigators validate the results of their nuclear investigations against contrast angiography - one cannot merely assume correlations achieved in other locations, even using the same methodology. Intra and inter-observer variation must be investigated also and all validations should be repeated should changes in method-ology be made.

The clinical uses of nuclear angiocardiography, shown in tables 4 and 5, are presented in detail later (Dymond, these Proceedings). Suffice it to say here that the main areas of clinical application lie in the early detection of ischaemic heart disease, the quantification of the extent of myocardial damage (eg following infarction) and the follow-up and assess-ment of both medical and surgical therapy. It will remain the method of choice for the non-invasive investigation of left and right ventricular function for the forseeable future.

6. Conclusion

In the short and medium term, there is no doubt that nuclear cardiology will play a major role in the practice of clinical cardiology. The pyrophosphate scan will continue to have a very limited application but the nuclear angiogram will remain the prime non-invasive method of assessing ventricular performance. In this area, ultrasonics has not yet proven reliable and, in a substantial number of patients, may never achieve reliability while intravenous digital subtraction angiography still requires the administration of large quantities of iodinated contrast material, gives poor quality data for patients with ejection fractions below 45% (Tobis et al., 1982) and suffers a severe cost dis-advantage (one can purchase five multicrystal gamma cameras for the cost of angiographic equipment). The investigation of myocardial perfusion and metabolism will continue, the expansion being pioneered by the positron-emitting radiopharmaceuticals: as "conventional" gamma-emitting analogues, such as the fatty acids, become available, more institutions will be able to perform these studies. Positron studies seem unlikely to be widely used on grounds of cost and seem destined to perform a valuable research role in a few major centres. Nuclear magnetic resonance is as yet untried in the clinical situation but, like X-ray computed tomography, suffers cost, availability and throughput limitations: at present, the time taken to produce images renders intervention studies difficult.

Given that the strength of nuclear medicine lies in its ability to study function (using minute quantities of a tracer) rather than to delineate anatomy, it is the field of myocardial perfusion/metabolism which will ensure the continuance of nuclear cardiology in the long term.

7. References

Abdullah AZ, Hawkins LA, Britton KE, Elliott AT and Stephens JD 1981
Nuc.Med.Commun. 2 268-277
Anger HO 1958 Rev.Sci.Instrum. 29 27
Beller GA and Pohost GM 1977 Circulation 56 141
Bender MA and Blau M 1962 Progress in Medical Radioisotope Scanning
(New York: USAEC)
Berger HJ, Davies RA, Batsford WP, Hoffer PB, Gottschalk A and Zaret BL
1981 Circulation 63 133-142
Berman DS, Staniloff H, Freeman M, Garcia E, Pantaleo N, Maddahi J,
Waxman A, Forrester J and Swan HJC 1980 Am.JCardiol. 45 481 (abst)
Bodenheimer MM, Banka VS, Fooshee C, Herman GA and Helfant RH 1978
Circulation 58 789-795
Bonte FJ, Parkey RW, Graham KD, Moore J and Stokely EM 1974 Radiology 110
473-474
Carr EA, Beierwaltes WI, Wengst AV and Barlett JD 1962 J.Nucl.Med. 3 76
Carr EA, Gleason G, Shaw J and Krontz B 1964 Am.Heart.J. 68 627
Conn HL 1962 Circ.Res. 10 505-515
Deutsch E, Libson K, Vandetheyden J-L, Nosco DL, Sodd VJ and Nishiyama H.
1982 J.Nucl.Med. 23 P9 (abst)
Donato L, Guintini C and Lewis ML 1962 Circulation 26 183-199
Dymond D, Stone D, Elliott AT, Britton KE, Banim SQ and Spurrell RAJ 1979
Br.Heart.J. 42 671-679
Dymond DS, Elliott AT, Stone D, Hendrix G and Spurrell RAJ 1982 Circulat-
ion 65 311-322
Ell PJ. Langford R, Pearce P, Lui D, Elliott AT, Woolf N and Williams ES
1978 Br.Heart.J. 40 226-233
Elliott AT, Dymond DS, Stone DL, Flatman W, Bett R, Cuninghame JG, Sims HE
and Willis HH 1983 Phys.Med.Biol. 28 i
Faris JV, Burt RW, Graham MC and Knowbel 5B 1982 Am.J.Cardiol. 49 733-742
Francisco DA, Collins SM, Go RT, Ehrahardt JC, van Kirk OC and Marcus ML
1982 Circulation 66 370-379
Freundlieb C, Hock A, Vyska K, Feinendegen LE, Machulla H-J and
Stocklin G 1980 J.Nucl.Med. 21 1043-1050
Green MV, Ostrow HG, Douglas MA, Myers RW, Scott RN, Bailey JJ and
Johnston GS 1975 J.Nucl.Med. 16 95-98
Gossman 2D, Foster AB, McAfee JG, Richardson R, Subramanian G, Markarian
B, Gagne G and Bassano D 1977 J.Nucl.Med. 18 51-56
Hamilton GW, Trobaugh GB, Ritchie JL, Gould KL, De Rouen TA and Williams
DL 1978 Sem.Nucl.Med. 8 358-364
Henze E, Schelbert HR, Barrio JR, Egbert JE, Hansen HW, MacDonald NS and
Phelps ME 1982 J.Nucl.Med. 23 671-681
Hoffman EJ, Phelps ME, Mullani NA, Higgins CS and Ter-Pogossian MM 1976
J.Nucl.Med. 17 493-503
Holman BL, Adams DF, Jewitt D, Eldh P, Idoine J, Cohn PF, Gorlin R and
Adelstein SJ 1974 Radiology 112 99-107
Holman BL, Friedman BJ, Polak JF, Curfman G, Wynne J, Kirsch C-M and
English RJ 1980 J.Nucl.Med. 21 P69 (abst)
Hurley PJ, Cooper M, Reba RC, Poggenburg KJ and Wagner HN 1971 J.Nucl.Med.
12 516-519
Jaszczak RJ, Murphy PH, Huard D and Burdine JA 1977 J.Nucl.Med. 18 373-
380
Keyes JW, Leonard PF, Brady SL, Svetkoff DJ, Rogers WL and Lucchesi BR
1978 Circulation 58 227-232
Kline RC, Swanson DP, Wieland DM, Thrall JH, Gross MD, Pitt B and
Beierwaltes WH 1981 J.Nucl.Med. 22 129-132
Kuhl DE and Edwards RQ 1963 Radiology 80 653-661

Leboeitz E, Greene MW, Bradley-Moore P, Atkins H, Ansari A, Richards P and Belgrave E 1973 J.Nucl.Med. 14 421-422 (abst)

Marshall RC, Berger HJ, Costin JC, Freedman GS, Wolberg J, Cohen LS, Gottschalk A and Zaret BL 1977 Circulation 56 820-829

Muchllehner G, Buchin MP and Dubek JH 1976 IEE Nucl.Sci. NS-23 528-537

Muller TM, Marcus ML, Ehrhardt JC, Chaudhuri T and Abboud FM 1976 Circulation 54 640-646

Murray RE, McKillop JH, Bessent RG, Turner JG, Lorimer HR, Hutton I, Greig WR and Lowrie TD 1979 Br.Heart.J. 41 568-574

Nielson A, Morris KG, Murdock RH, Bruno FP and Cobb FR 1979 Circulation 59-60 Supp II - 148 (abst)

Olson HG, Lyons KP, Aronow LS, Kupetus J, Orlando J and Hughes D 1979 Am.J.Cardiol. 43 889-898

Otto CA, Brown LE, Wieland DM and Beierwaltes WH 1981 J.Nucl.Med 22 613-18

Pavel DG, Zimmer AM and Patterson VN 1977 J.Nucl.Med. 18 305 308

Parkey RW, Bonte FJ, Buja LM, Stokely EM and Willerson JT 1977 Sem.Nucl.Med. 7 15-28

Pfisterer ME, Ricci DR, Schuler G, Swanson SS, Gordon DG, Peterson KE and Ashburn WL 1979 J.Nucl.Med. 20 484-490

Phelps ME, Hoffman EJ, Selin C, Huang S-C, Robinson G, MacDonald N, Schelbert H and Kuhl DE 1978 J.Nucl.Med. 19 1311-1319

Pitt B and Strauss HW 1976 Am.J.Cardiol. 37 797-806

Pohost GM, Zir LM, Moor RH, McKusik KA, Guiney TE and Beller GA 1977 Circulation 55 294-302

Prinzmetal M, Corday E, Bergman HC, Schwarz L and Spritzler RJ 1948 Science 108 340-341

Ratib O, Phelps ME, Juang S-C, Henze E, Selin CE and Schnelbert HR 1982 J.Nucl.Med. 22 577-586

Ritchie JL, Hamilton GW, Williams DL and Kennedy JW 1976 Radiology 121 131-138

Roberts R, Sobel BE and Parker CW 1978 Clin.Chim.Acta. 83 141

Royal HD, Brown PH and Claunch BC 1979 J.Nucl.Med. 20 977-980

Selwyn AP, Forse G, Fox KM and Steiner R 1980 Br.Heart.J. 43 112 (abst)

Shell WE, Kligerman M, Rorke P and Burnam M 1979 Am.J.Cardiol. 44 67-75

Smith TD, and Richards P 1976 J.Nucl.Med. 17 126-132

Stokely EM, Tipton M, Buja LM, Lewis SE, De Vous M, Bonte FJ, Parkey RW and Willerson JT 1979 Circulation 59-60 Supp II - 27 (abst)

Tobis J, Nacioglu O, Johnston WD, Siebert A, Iseri LT, Roeck W, Elkayam U and Henry WL 1982 Am.Heart.J. 104 20-27

Vogel RA, Kirch DL, Lefree MT, Rainwater JO, Jensen DP and Steele PP 1979 Am.J.Cardiol. 43 787-793

Wackers FJ, Sokile EB, Samson G, van der Schoot JB, Lie KI, Lien KL and Wellens HJJ 1976 N.Engl.J.Med. 295 1-5

Wagner HN, Wake R, Nickoloff E and Natarajan TK 1976 Am.J.Cardiol. 38 747-750

Weiss ES, Ahmed SA, Welch MJ, Williamson JR, Ter-Pogossian MM and Sobel BE 1977 Circulation 55 66-73

Welch MJ, Thakur ML, Coleman RE, Patel M, Siegel BA and Ter-Pogossian MM 1977 J.Nucl.Med. 18 558-562

Wieland DM, Brown LE, Rogers WL, Worthington KC, Wu J-I, Clinthorne NH, Otto CA, Swanson DP and Beierwaltes WH 1981 J.Nucl.Med. 22 22-31

Willerson JT, Parkey RW, Bonte FJ, Meyer SL, Atkins JM and Stokely EM 1975 Circulation 51 1046-1052

Wong DW, Dhawan VK, Tanaka T, Mishkin FS, Reese IC and Thadepalli H 1982 J.Nucl.Med. 23 229-234

Myocardial Perfusion: Thallium and Beyond

J H McKillop

University Department of Medicine,
Royal Infirmary, Glasgow, G4 0SF.

Summary.   Myocardial imaging with the monovalent cation thallium-201 provides a non-invasive method of assessing myocardial perfusion. This review discusses the clinical utility of the technique and indicates that its main role is in the assessment of patients in whom there is some doubt about a diagnosis of coronary artery disease. Thallium-201 is not an ideal radiopharmaceutical and this has stimulated a search for an alternative myocardial imaging agent. The present status of iodine-123 labelled fatty acids as myocardial imaging agents is considered and preliminary data on a promising new technetium-99m labelled compound is briefly summarised.

1. Introduction

Scintigraphic assessment of myocardial perfusion can be carried out either by invasive or by non-invasive methods. The invasive techniques require the injection of radiolabelled macro-aggregates of albumin or radioactive inert gases directly into the coronary arteries at catheter-isation. The non-invasive studies utilise the intravenous administration of a variety of radiopharmaceuticals which actively accumulate within the myocardium. The invasive methods have largely research rather than routine clinical application and will not be discussed in this paper. The main non-invasive method currently available is thallium-201 (Tl201) imaging. This has been widely employed since the introduction of the substance by Lebowitz and colleagues in 1975, though some authorities still question the usefulness of Tl201 imaging (Burch 1980). The aim of the present review will be to summarise the clinical utility of this technique. Because Tl201 has properties which make it less than ideal as a radiopharmaceutical, the search continues for a better myocardial imaging agent and some of the newer compounds will be considered.

2. Thallium-201 Myocardial Imaging

2.1   Theoretical considerations and techniques

In 1964 Carr and colleagues reported the successful imaging of the human heart using a rectilinear scanner and the intravenous administration of the potassium analogue caesium-131 (Carr et al, 1964). They were able to identify sites of myocardial infarction as areas of reduced isotope uptake. Various potassium analogues were introduced in the next 10 years, but a widely applicable myocardial agent became available only with the introduction of Tl201 (Lebowitz et al, 1975). Though belonging to a

different group of the periodic table from potassium, Tl is able to
substitute for potassium in the ATP-ase dependent sodium-potassium pump
situated in the membrane of active cells (Mullins and Moore, 1960;
Gehring and Hammond, 1967). Following intravenous injection, Tl201 is
widely distributed in the body (Strauss et al, 1975) with approximately
4% of the injected dose accumulating in the heart (Strauer et al, 1978).
Various drugs, notably digoxin, may alter Tl201 uptake in vitro, but in
clinical studies such drugs do not seem to affect the quality of the image
obtained (Hamilton et al, 1978).

The extraction of Tl201 on first pass through the coronary circulation is
around 80% (Strauss et al, 1975) so that maximal myocardial uptake is
achieved rapidly. The main determinant of myocardial uptake in clinical
practice is regional myocardial perfusion. Under conditions of reduced
flow myocardial uptake of Tl201 is linearly related to perfusion, but
coronary hyperaemia produces a less than expected augmentation of tracer
uptake (Strauss et al, 1975). The uptake of Tl201 by the myocardium is
also dependent on an intact sodium-potassium pump and any abnormality of
myocardial metabolism can impair Tl201 uptake. Thus a Tl201 image defect
is not specific for coronary artery disease. Some evidence suggests that
Tl201 image defects appear in coronary artery disease only when the
reduction in flow is sufficiently severe to cause myocardial ischaemia,
that is, disrupts myocardial metabolism (Selwyn et al, 1978).

Thallium-201 has a physical half-life of 73.5 hours. The emissions used
for imaging are 69-83 keV X-rays derived from a mercury daughter. The
low energy of the X-rays causes some problems with tissue attenuation
and with reduced intrinsic resolution compared to technetium-99m
(McKillop, 1982). The radiation dose associated with Tl201 imaging has
been estimated at 0.24 rads/mCi for the whole body and 1.2 rads/mCi for
the kidney, the critical organ (Lebowitz et al, 1975; Atkins et al, 1977).
Because of this radiation dosimetry, the injected dose of Tl201 is usually
limited to 2 mCi in patient studies, resulting in a relatively low count
rate from the myocardium. This is further complicated by the poor target
to background activity ratio, typically around 2/1 for heart/lung on rest
studies (Hamilton et al, 1978). Visualisation of the inferior myocardium
can be obscured by uptake in upper abdominal organs, especially on
resting studies. Splanchnic uptake can be reduced by studying the patient
in a fasting state (Atkins et al, 1977).

Imaging studies can be carried out with any modern gamma camera. The energy
analyser   of the camera is centred on 80 keV with a 20% window.
Multiple projections, typically anterior, one or more left anterior
oblique and a left lateral image are obtained, as different areas of the
left ventricular are best seen in each view (McKillop, 1982). Most
projections are obtained with the patient supine, but it is recommended
that the left lateral is performed with the patient lying on his right
side, as this reduces the likelihood of diaphragmatic attenuation of the
emissions producing a false positive abnormality in the infero-posterior
area (Johnstone et al, 1979). Refinements   the acquisition process such
as 7-pinhole tomographic imaging or ECG gating do not significantly
increase the accuracy (Berman et al,1980; McKillop et al, 1981).

Thallium-201 imaging may be carried out after injecting the tracer at rest
or during stress, typically a symptom limited exercise test. The normal
myocardial image is horseshoe or doughnut shaped, corresponding to
homogeneous activity in the left ventricular wall with a central colder

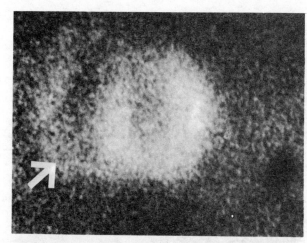

Figure 1

Normal unprocessed
stress 30 LAO Tl201
image. Note both left
ventricular and right
ventricular (arrow)
visualisation.

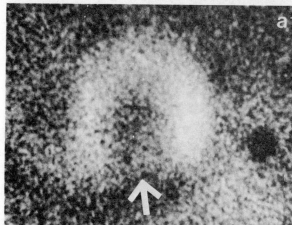

Figure 2

30 LAO Tl201 images at
stress (a) and rest
(b) showing fixed
apico inferior defect
(arrow) due to prior
infarction.

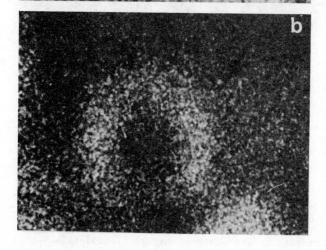

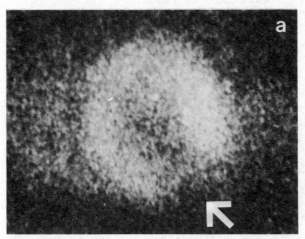

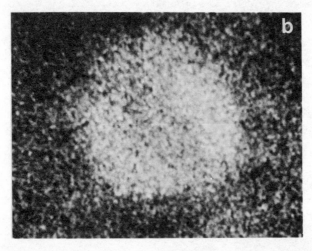

Figure 3

30 LAO Tl201 images at
stress (a) and rest (b)
showing reversible apico
inferior defect (arrow)
due to myocardial
ischaemia from right
coronary artery disease.

area due to the ventricular cavity (Cook et al, 1976). The right
ventricle is frequently seen on stress studies (Fig. 1) but not on rest
studies unless there is right ventricular hypertrophy (Khaja et al, 1979).
Injecting during stress is important because, unless myocardial infarction
has occurred, myocardial blood flow at rest remains normal distal to a
coronary artery stenosis until it occupies more than 90% of the luminal
diameter (Gould and Lipscomb, 1974). By contrast, the increase in
myocardial blood flow induced by stress is impaired distal to coronary
stenoses of 50% or more. By comparing the findings on rest and stress
images it is possible to classify Tl201 image abnormalities as either
fixed (present on both rest and stress studies) or reversible (present
only at stress). A fixed defect at rest (Fig. 2) usually implies the
presence of myocardial scar. It may be due to myocardial infarction but
many other processes, for example cardiomyopathy or space occupying
lesions of the myocardium such as sarcoidosis, may also cause fixed

defects. Reversible defects present at exercise and absent at rest (Fig.3) indicate the presence of impaired but viable myocardium and are usually due to myocardial ischaemia. Reversible defects are more specific for coronary artery disease than fixed defects.

When carrying out post stress imaging it is important to complete acquisition as soon as possible after injection, as ischaemic defects tend to "fill in" with the passage of time due to redistribution of Tl201. It has recently been suggested that as many as 15% of stress induced abnormalities may disappear within 30 minutes of injection(Makler et al 1982) The property of redistribution of Tl201 into ischaemic areas has been used in the technique of delayed imaging (Pohost et al, 1977), whereby a standard stress Tl201 study is followed by repeat imaging 4 to 6 hours later without injecting any more radioisotope. This method usually allows the differentiation between fixed and reversible defects to be made with a single injection of radiopharmaceutical, thus reducing the patient's radiation exposure and the cost of the study. Though redistribution images usually show some reversibility of the defect when myocardial ischaemia is present, thus allowing this diagnosis to be made, they tend to overestimate the fixed component present (Ritchie et al, 1979). Therefore, in situations where an accurate estimate of the extent of myocardial scarring is required, rest images are probably preferable to redistribution studies.

Thallium-201 myocardial images may be analysed visually, with or without computer processing. Simple background subtraction and contrast enhancement tend to improve sensitivity at the cost of reduced specificity (McKillop et al, 1980). This shortcoming may be improved by interpolative background subtraction (Goris et al, 1976). Quantitative analysis, either by deriving count densities for different myocardial areas (McKillop et al, 1980) or by more sophisticated techniques of plotting regional Tl201 washout over several hours (Berman et al, 1980) appear to have greater accuracy than visual analysis.

2.2   Clinical results

Rest Tl201 images often demonstrate abnormalities in patients with myocardial infarction. Wackers and colleagues have shown that if patients are studied within 6 hours of the onset of chest pain a normal Tl201 image effectively excludes an acute infarct and thus can be used reliably in deciding that a patient does not require admission to the coronary care unit (Wackers et al, 1979). There are, however, not inconsiderable problems in using Tl201 in acute infarction. Firstly there must be constant availability of the radiopharmaceutical. Secondly, it is not possible to study many patients within 6 hours of the onset of symptoms and false negative studies become increasingly frequent with the passage of time (Wackers et al, 1976; McKillop et al, 1978). Even if an abnormal image is obtained in a patient with chest pain, it is not possible to say whether the abnormality represents acute infarction, old infarction, acute myocardial ischaemia or some other pathological process unrelated to ischaemic heart disease (McKillop et al, 1978). For these various reasons Tl201 imaging has little role in the patient with suspected acute myocardial infarction. The technique produces more promising results in assessing the prognosis of patients recently recovered from acute infarction, with both rest (Gibson et al, 1980) and stress (Turner et al, 1980) imaging apparently being able to identify groups of patients who are at high risk of an early recurrent event and thus merit angiographic study with a view to coronary artery surgery.

The main clinical use of Tl201 imaging has been in the study of patients with suspected myocardial ischaemia. Many studies have now been published in the literature comparing Tl201 imaging to coronary arteriography and several recent reviews are available (McKillop, 1982; Berger and Zaret, 1981; Berman et al 1980). Stress Tl201 imaging when analysed with computer processing of images or by a quantitative technique shows a sensitivity of between 80% and 90% for the detection of significant coronary artery disease and a specificity of 85% to 95%. Series comparing Tl201 imaging to stress electrocardiography have almost invariably shown both higher sensitivity and specificity for the scintigraphic technique. Studies in patients with single vessel disease have correlated areas on the Tl201 image with individual vessel territories. As might be expected there is considerable overlap in the right and left circumflex coronary artery territories (Dunn et al, 1980). As a result of this and other factors such as differing severity of individual stenoses and the presence of collateral vessels, stress Tl201 imaging frequently underestimates the extent of disease in patients with multivessel disease and cannot be relied on to identify this high risk group (McKillop et al, 1979; Rigo et al, 1980).

Because of lack of perfect sensitivity and inability to identify reliably patients with multivessel disease, Tl201 imaging is not recommended in patients who have typical angina pectoris (Hamilton, 1979; Sisson, 1981). The main clinical application of the technique is in the evaluation of patients in whom the diagnosis of coronary artery disease is less certain on clinical grounds, such as those with atypical chest pain, those with equivocal or non-diagnostic stress ECG's or asymptomatic individuals with a positive stress ECG. In each of these situations, which are clinically very difficult, Tl201 imaging is extremely useful in deciding on the need to proceed to invasive investigations. Because of low diagnostic yield, expense and radiation exposure, Tl201 imaging is not advised for screening asymptomatic populations (McKillop, 1982; Hamilton, 1979).

The value of Tl201 imaging in the assessment of patients who have undergone coronary artery bypass grafting is more controversial (McKillop, 1982; Berman et al, 1980). While some studies have shown a good correlation between stress Tl201 image appearances and the patency of bypass grafts as judged by postoperative coronary angiography, other workers have found that there is a significant incidence of normal myocardial images in patients with occluded grafts. If an area that is abnormal on the preoperative stress Tl201 study becomes normal on an adequate stress test postoperatively, then it is likely that the graft is patent. Conversely, an area which is normal preoperatively but abnormal at a similar work load postoperatively implies either graft occlusion or progression of native disease. If no change is observed in a region on the pre and postoperative images, it is not possible to comment on the adequacy of revascularisation of that area.

Thallium-201 imaging has proven valuable in a variety of other cardiac conditions. Patients with mitral valve prolapse and chest pain usually show Tl201 image abnormalities only if there is also coronary disease (Massie et al, 1978). Thallium-201 imaging can be used to demonstrate a reversible reduction in myocardial perfusion during episodes of coronary artery spasm (Maseri et al, 1976) and may be of value in assessing the

functional significance of a borderline lesion seen at arteriography
(Berman et al, 1980). In patients with cardiomyopathy Tl201 images can be
used to screen for right ventricular hypertrophy and a characteristic scan
appearance has been described in hypertrophic subaortic stenosis (Bulkley
et al, 1975). Thallium-201 imaging is disappointing in patients with
aortic valvular stenosis with both false positive studies in patients who
do not have coronary disease, and false negative studies in some with
coronary disease (Bailey et al, 1977).

3. Labelled Fatty Acid Imaging

As discussed above, for reasons of physical characteristics, physiological
factors, radiation dosimetry and cost, while Tl201 is often clinically
useful, it is not an ideal myocardial imaging agent. The search,
therefore, continues for a better radiopharmaceutical and at present the
most promising group are the radiolabelled fatty acids.

In 1965, Evans and his colleagues showed that scintigraphic images of the
heart could be obtained after injecting iodine-131 (I131) labelled oleic
acid, prepared by double bond saturation (Evans et al, 1965). However,
I131 is not very suitable for gamma-camera imaging, and is associated with
a high radiation dose. Additionally, the method of radioiodination alters
the properties of the compound sufficiently to reduce myocardial extraction
compared to "natural" compounds such as Carbon-11 (C11) labelled palmitate
(Robinson and Lee, 1975). While C11 labelled compounds are very
efficiently extracted by the myocardium, the necessity for a nearby
cyclotron because of the 20 minute half-life and the requirement for
special equipment to image the positrons emitted make it unlikely they
will be widely used as myocardial imaging agents in the foreseeable future.
Recently, however, it has been shown that long chain fatty acids, labelled
in the terminal (omega) position have extraction efficiencies similar
to C11 palmitate (Machulla et al, 1978), while the substitution of I123
for I131 has improved both imaging characteristics and radiation dosimetry.
The physiological properties of the I123 labelled long chain fatty acids
vary according to the chain length with highest extraction being reported
for those with chains of 18 to 21 carbon atoms (Otto et al, 1981). The
fatty acids being most widely investigated in clinical practice at present
are I123 hexadecanoic acid (16 carbon chain) and I123 heptadecanoic acid
(17 carbon chain). The precise metabolic characteristics of these two
compounds are not yet clear, but it seems possible that they do not differ
significantly when studied in patients (Van der Wall et al, 1981 a).

Following intravenous injection, I123 labelled free fatty acids (I123 FFA)
are rapidly taken up by myocardium with approximately 4% of the
administered dose accumulating in the myocardium (Otto et al, 1981). The
distribution of I123 FFA in the myocardium is proportional to myocardial
blood flow as judged by Tl201 uptake (Westera et al, 1980). The labelled
fatty acid is then thought to be metabolised by the myocardial cells by
β oxidation. In myocardial ischaemia this metabolic pathway is impaired.
Thus areas of myocardial ischaemia are characterised on I123 FFA imaging
by reduced accumulation of the tracer and by slower than normal metabolism
of that which is taken up (Freundlieb et al, 1980).

Following injection of the tracer, imaging should begin within 5 minutes
(Freundlieb et al, 1980). With time, metabolism of the FFA releases free
I123 into the blood resulting in an increase in background counts so that
acceptable images are not usually obtained more that 30 minutes after

administration. This allows adequate time to perform a four view study if the standard dose of 1-3 mCi of the radiopharmaceutical is administered. Images can then be analysed visually. An alternative method of study is to obtain only an LAO image and calculate the regional washout of activity from the myocardium using a method of correction for background (non-cardiac) activity (Freundlieb et al, 1980).

Relatively few studies are as yet available of the clinical application of I123 FFA myocardial imaging. Comparison of T1201 and I123 FFA images at rest or after stress injections generally shows good correlation between the regional distribution of the two radiopharmaceuticals, though some exceptions are found (Van der Wall et al, 1980; Abdullah et al, 1981). The significance of differing distributions is not known. When regional washout curves are obtained after stress injection of the radio-pharmaceutical, areas of myocardial ischaemia have a washout half-time significantly prolonged beyond the normal mean value of around 25 minutes (Vyska et al, 1979; Van der Wall et al, 1981 b). It is theoretically possible that quantitation of regional washout in this fashion will allow more accurate prediction of multivessel disease than has proved possible with T1201. A recent study suggests that infarcted and ischaemic areas differ when the washout is calculated on a stress I123 FFA study, with the infarcted region showing a shorter than normal half-time (Van der Wall et al, 1981 a).

Validation involving large scale clinical trials is required for I123 labelled free fatty acids and it will be necessary to elucidate what information about myocardial metabolism can be gained by imaging with fatty acids of differing chain lengths. Further work is also necessary on reliable production of a pure and stable radiopharmaceutical. Labelled fatty acid myocardial imaging, however, does hold great promise of becoming a clinically valuable tool in the assessment of patients with suspected or established coronary artery disease.

4. Other Myocardial Imaging Agents

Nitrogen-13 ammonia is accumulated by the myocardium by a method similar to the potassium analogues, and can demonstrate cold spots due to myocardial ischaemia or infarction (Harper et al, 1973). However, as with C11 labelled fatty acids, the short half-life, cyclotron production and positron emissions make it unsuitable for general use. A number of other labelled metabolites such as β blocker analogues, bretylium analogues, nitrogen-13 asparaginase and toluidine blue analogues have undergone some evaluation as myocardial imaging agents (Mills et al, 1981) but as yet they have yielded no radiopharmaceutical which is suitable for clinical use.

Considerable effort has been made to find a myocardial imaging agent which can be labelled with technetium-99m (Tc99m). Such a compound would have ideal imaging characteristics for the gamma camera, low radiation dose and, if a kit could be produced, would be available at any time in every nuclear medicine department. Various cationic complexes have been assessed (Deutsch et al, 1981). Of this group of compounds Tc99m-dimethylphosphino ethane (DMPE) shows considerable promise (Deutsch et al, 1981; Thakur, 1982). Studies of Tc99m-DMPE myocardial distribution at rest suggest it correlates with regional blood flow even better than T1201 and animal data indicate it may be a potentially useful agent for the study of ischaemic heart disease (Nishiyama et al, 1982). Should these early promising results be confirmed, then Tc99m-DMPE will be a most exciting method for evaluating myocardial perfusion non-invasively.

References

Abdullah A Z, Hawkins L A, Britton K E et al 1981 Nucl. Med. Comm. 5 268
Atkins H L, Budinger T F, Lebowitz E et al 1977 J. Nucl. Med. 18 133
Bailey I K, Come P C, Kelly D T et al 1977 Am. J. Cardiol 40 889
Berger H J and Zaret B L 1981 N. Engl. J. Med. 305 799
Berman D, Freeman M, Garcia E et al 1980 J. Nucl. Med. 21 70
Berman D S, Garcia E V and Maddahi J 1980 Nuclear Medicine Annual 1980
    eds L M Freeman and H S Weissmann (New York: Raven) pp 1-56
Bulkley B H, Rouleau J, Strauss H W et al 1975 N. Engl. J. Med. 293 1113
Burch G E, 1980 Am. Heart J. 99 540
Carr E A, Gleason G, Shaw J et al 1964 Am. Heart J. 68 627
Cook D J, Bailey I, Strauss H W et al 1976 J. Nucl. Med. 17 583
Deutsch E, Glavan K A, Sodd V J et al 1981 J. Nucl. Med. 22 897
Dunn R F, Freedman B, Bailey I K et al 1980 J. Nucl. Med. 21 717
Evans J R, Gunton R W, Baker R G et al 1965 Circ. Res. 16 1
Freundlieb C, Hock A, Vyska K et al 1980 J. Nucl. Med. 21 1043
Gehring P J and Hammond P B 1967 J. Pharm. Exp. Ther. 155 187
Gibson R S, Taylor G J, Watson D D et al 1980 J. Nucl. Med. 21 1015
Goris M L, Daspit S G, McLaughlin P et al 1976 J. Nucl. Med. 17 744
Gould K L and Lipscomb K 1974 Am. J. Cardiol. 34 48
Hamilton G W 1979 J. Nucl. Med. 20 1201
Hamilton G W, Narahara K A, Yee H et al 1978 J. Nucl. Med. 19 10
Harper P V, Schwartz T, Beck R N et al 1973 Radiology 108 613
Johnstone D E, Wackers F J, Berger H J et al 1979 J. Nucl. Med. 20 183
Khaja F, Alam M, Goldstein S et al 1979 Circulation 59 182
Lebowitz E, Greene M W, Fairchild R et al 1975 J. Nucl. Med. 16 151
Machulla H J, Stocklin G, Kupfernagel C H et al 1978 J. Nucl. Med. 19 298
Makler P T, Alavi A, McCarthy D M et al 1982 J. Nucl. Med. 23 P19
Maseri A, Parodi D, Saveri S et al 1976 Circulation 54 280
Massie B, Botvinick E H, Shames D et al 1978 Circulation 57 19
McKillop J H 1982 CRC Crit. Rev. Diag. Imag. (in press)
McKillop J H, Fawcett M D, Baumert J E et al 1981 J. Nucl. Med. 22 219
McKillop J H, Gray H W, Turner J G et al 1978 Br. Heart J. 40 870
McKillop J H, Murray R G, Turner J G et al 1979 J. Nucl. Med. 20 715
McKillop J H, Murray R G, Turner J G et al 1980 Radiology 136 187
Mills S L, Basmadjian G P and Ice R D 1981 J. Pharm. Sci. 70 1
Mullins L J and Moore R D 1960 J. Gen. Physiol. 43 759
Nishiyama H, Sodd V J, Deutsch E A et al 1982 J. Nucl. Med. 23 P12
Otto C A, Brown L E, Wieland D M et al 1981 J. Nucl. Med. 22 613
Pohost G M, Zir L M, Moore R H et al 1977 Circulation 55 294
Rigo P, Bailey I K, Griffith L S C et al 1980 Circulation 61 973
Ritchie J L, Albro P C, Caldwell J H et al 1979 J. Nucl. Med. 20 477
Robinson G D and Lee A W 1975 J. Nucl. Med. 16 17
Selwyn A P, Welmann E, Pratt T et al 1978 Circ. Res. 43 287
Sisson J C 1981 J. Nucl. Med. 22 303
Strauss H W, Harrison K, Langan J K et al 1975 Circulation 51 641
Strauer B E, Burger S and Bull U 1978 Bas. Res. Cardiol. 73 298
Thakur M L 1982 J. Nucl. Med. 23 P11
Turner J D, Schwartz K M, Logic J R et al 1980 Circulation 61 729

Van der Wall E E, Heidendal G A K, Hollander W et al 1980
    Eur. J. Nucl. Med. 5 401
Van der Wall E E, Heidendal G A K, Hollander W et al 1981 a
    Eur. J. Nucl. Med. 6 383
Van der Wall E E, Heidendal G A K, Hollander W et al 1981 b
    Eur. J. Nucl. Med. 6 391
Vyska K, Hock A, Profant M et al 1979 J. Nucl. Med. 20 650
Wackers F J, Sokole E B, Samson G et al 1976 N. Engl. J. Med. 295 1
Wackers F J, Lie K I, Liem K L et al 1979 Br. Heart J. 41 111
Westera G, Van der Wall E E, Heidendal G A K et al 1980
    Eur. J. Nucl. Med. 5 339

First Pass and Equilibrium Measurements of Ventricular Function

D S Dymond

Cardiac Department, St. Bartholomew's Hospital, London EC1A 7BE.

1. Introduction

Dynamic imaging of the heart using radiopharmaceuticals has now become almost as routine in some cardiac centres as echocardiography or Holter monitoring. The unique properties of radio-tracers, and the ease with which they may be administered by peripheral venous injections, make them attractive as a means for studying left and right heart function repeatedly and longitudinally. This is not practicable with contrast angiography which is not only invasive but carries a measurable risk. The sophisticated imaging equipment and powerful computers now in use have enabled us not only to study the heart on a chamber-by-chamber basis, but also to examine different regions inside a chamber in some detail. In this review, the different methods available for dynamic cardiac studies will be discussed, along with their strengths and weaknesses, and clinical utility.

2. First pass studies

By definition, such studies involve the acquisition of dynamic data for the short time (30-50 seconds) needed for the intravenously injected tracer to pass through the central circulation. One of the first such studies was carried out by Prinzmetal et al (1948) who produced a double-peaked curve of tracer passage through right and left heart chambers and coined the term "radiocardiogram". Current first pass studies differ from this inasmuch as they are displayed not only as curves, but also as images that provide information on the anatomical and spatial distribution of the tracer. From these images it is possible to identify the individual cardiac chambers and to generate time-activity curves from them. The curves may be displayed as radiocardiograms to allow calculation of cardiac output, pulmonary transit times or intracardiac shunts (Jones et al 1972), or as high frequency curves from individual chambers in order to visualise the cyclical fluctuations of counts within individual cardiac cycles. The peaks and troughs of these curves represent end-diastoles and end-systoles respectively. As counts within a chamber are directly proportional to the volume of that chamber at any one time, then the changes in count density may be used to calculate changes in relative chamber volume (Marshall et al 1977, Dymond et al 1979).

The technical requirements in order for first pass studies to be reliable are as follows:
1) The activity should be injected as a bolus of 15-20 mCi contained in as small a volume as possible, i.e. with high specific activity. The Tc-99m does not need to be bound to an intravascular marker such as red

cells as it only has to remain in the vascular space for 30-50 seconds. Hence, free pertechnetate is acceptable. The small bolus does aid in temporal separation of the cardiac chambers, which is mandatory for successful first pass studies. Reproducibility of data is also closely related to bolus integrity (Dymond et al 1982a). The bolus must be injected with a rapid 20cc saline flush.

2) As the diastoles and systoles are apparent from the individual curves of each chamber as the isotope passes through, it is unnecessary to record an ECG signal to identify the phases of the cardiac cycle. The studies are "intrinsically gated". However, there must be enough frames of data per cardiac cycle in order to avoid blurring the cycle and assigning, for example, early diastolic elements to a frame labelled end-systole. This requires at least 20 frames/second for resting studies and 30 frames/second for exercise.

3) The count density must be adequate. As there is only a short time available for data acquisition, and there are only a few (5-10) cardiac cycles involved in the first pass, the maximum information must be accumulated in order to obtain enough counts for the study to be statistically reliable. This requires instruments with high count-rate capabilities. At present the multicrystal camera is the best instrument to achieve this, with count-rates in excess of 350,000 counts/second.

The count-rates of single crystal instruments are increasing, and such cameras are now more suitable for first pass studies (Flatman et al 1983). Assuming good temporal resolution, the reliability of numerical information and functional images is related to the information density (Walton et al 1980). There are ways of improving first pass statistics, such as summation of individual cycles to produce a representative cycle with high counts, or temporal smoothing of dynamic data to improve signal-to-noise ratio (Dymond et al 1982b).

3.Equilibrium studies

Unlike the first pass studies in which the cardiac chambers are separated temporally, the equilibrium blood-pool technique requires that a tracer be allowed to equilibrate within the entire vascular space for 3 to 5 minutes after injection, prior to imaging. The radiopharmaceutical must remain within the vascular compartment, and Tc-99m is usually tagged to the patients' own red blood cells to achieve this. Red cells provide a superior blood-pool marker to human serum albumin which tends to leak from the vascular space, and also to be denatured during radio-labelling, which leads to accumulation in the liver. As all cardiac chambers contain activity at the same time, and as only a small fraction of the injected dose is in the heart at equilibrium, "extrinsic gating" is required to identify the phases of the cardiac cycle. The usual such gating signal is the ECG, which is used to control the time intervals during which data are collected. Originally, end-systolic and end-diastolic gating only were performed (Strauss et al 1971) but this has now been superceded by multi-gated acquisition techniques or M.U.G.A. (Burow et al 1977) whereby the cardiac cycle is divided into sequential frames of equal duration. Each frame may be only of 30-50 milliseconds duration, and as there are insufficient counts in any one frame to produce adequate statistics, data are collected and integrated over several hundred cardiac cycles. The short time available for first pass acquisition is therefore not a limitation of this technique, and similarly, count-rate capabilities are not a problem as they may be overcome simply by prolongation of the data acquisition time. Because of the importance of the ECG signal in data acquisition, it is vital to monitor significant changes in heart rate as such changes will distort the frame relationships in the cardiac cycle. The presence of multiple ectopic beats or of atrial fibrillation will cause such distortions. Fortunately, because data acquisition time is not limited, "unacceptable" beats may be rejected without compromising statistics. It is apparent that multi-gated studies do not require specialised high count-rate equipment but may be carried out on standard single crystal cameras interfaced to a computer. The relationship between counts and volume naturally applies equally well to these studies.

4.Comparison of first pass and equilibrium studies

There is continuing debate on which of the techniques is superior but in the final analysis the information obtainable is largely identical, although the first pass method does allow shunt detection and calculation of transit times as well as assessment of ventricular function. Each technique does have particular strengths and weaknesses which must be considered when choosing which to apply to a given clinical problem. A detailed comparison may be found elsewhere (Thrall et al 1980, Knapp et al 1981), and some of the important differences in terms of imaging equipment and radiopharmaceuticals have been discussed above. The major advantages of the first pass technique are:-
1) Flexibility of projection, particularly the ability to use the RAO view. The equilibrium method is limited to use of the LAO view to separate right and left ventricles. This is not the optimal projection to assess regional left ventricular function. The straight anterior view may be used if the right heart is not unduly dilated but the RAO usually leads to superimposition of right ventricular activity over the inferior and septal parts of the left ventricle.
2) The short data acquisition time which makes the first pass method attractive for exercise studies as patients may be taken to true "end-point". With gated imaging times of approximately 2 minutes, it is difficult to obtain peak exercise studies. Many equilibrium users have tried alternative stress tests such as isometric hand grip or the cold pressor test which do not have sudden end-points, although the success of these has been variable (Wynne et al 1981, Manyari et al 1982).

Major disadvantages of the first pass technique are:-
1) The necessity for a separate injection of radionuclide for each sequential study or view. This of course limits the number of studies that can be performed, as radiation dosages rapidly accumulate.The development of new, short-lived radiopharmaceuticals such as gold-195m with a half-life of only 30.5 seconds is helping to overcome this limitation (Elliott et al 1983, Dymond et al 1983) but as yet the availability of gold-195m is limited.
2) Analysis of left ventricular function which depends on the function of the right ventricle being sufficiently good to eject the bolus compactly enough to allow separation of right from left heart. In patients with severely compromised right ventricular function or tricuspid regurgitation,first pass studies may not be possible via peripheral venous injections. Under those circumstances the choice rests between a first pass study performed via a central injection (Swan-Ganz catheter) or an equilibrium study in the LAO view.
3) Rejection of ectopic or post-ectopic beats likely to lead to poor statistics, as there are only a limited number of beats available in the first pass. As outlined above, this is not a problem with gated studies,

especially as most computers can be programmed to reject beats falling
outside a preset acceptable cycle length.
The major single advantage of the multiple gated acquisition method is
the ability to perform multiple studies over a period of hours after a
single tracer injection.

5.Measurement of left ventricular ejection fraction

Left ventricular ejection fraction has probably been the single most
measured index of cardiac performance using radioisotopic techniques.
There is little doubt that the ejection fraction is one of the most
useful such measurements, being intimately related to prognosis or
predicted operative mortality (Cohn et al 1974). The exact method for
determining ejection fraction depends on the mode of data acquisition. In
the early days of equilibrium imaging, where only analog images were
available, ejection fraction was calculated from the radionuclide images
using the area-length method for contrast angiograms applied to the image
contours (Strauss et al 1971). This has the disadvantage of making the
same assumptions about the conformity of the left ventricle to a
particular shape as does contrast angiography. Currently, with modern
computer power, calculations exploit the unique relationship between
activity in a chamber and the volume of that chamber at each point in the
cardiac cycle (Parker et al 1972). Thus ejection fraction is computed
as
(end diastolic counts-end systolic counts)/(end diastolic counts-
background counts).
The steps involved in this calculation are the generation of a region of
interest over the left ventricle and production of a time-activity curve
from that chamber. The curve includes counts from background, extra-
ventricular regions, and a correction for this background is therefore
mandatory and a crucial step in the calculations. For first pass studies,
where background in right heart, lungs and left atrium changes with time
as the activity washes out of those structures into the left ventricle,
corrections are time-dependent. Most workers have used a modification of
the method of Van Dyke et al (1972) but others have used a matrix of
activity in lung and left atrium to correct (Marshall et al 1977, Dymond
et al 1982b). A full discussion of the various corrections available is
beyond the scope of this article, but many reported studies have
testified to the good agreement between contrast angiographic ejection
fraction and radionuclide values (Van Dyke et al 1972, Schelbert et al
1975, Marshall et al 1977, Dymond et al 1982b). For gated studies,
background corrections are not time dependent as the activity in
background structures is at equilibrium. Usually, a horse-shoe shaped
area just outside the left ventricle is selected and background counts
per channel subtracted from the left ventricular curve. If the changes in
regional background activity are relatively homogeneous then an
interpolative correction may be more accurate than simple averaging
(Goris et al 1976). Again, the values obtained from these studies agree
closely with contrast angiographic measurements (Burow et al 1977,
Folland et al 1977, Wackers et al 1979)and the use of semi-automatic
techniques minimises inter-observer variability (Burow et al 1977,
Wackers et al 1979).

It must be remembered that radionuclide and contrast ejection fractions
are never likely to agree perfectly. Large differences may occur
particularly in diseased, distorted ventricles whose shape deviates from

the prolate spheroid model required for the area-length formulae. In
these cases the geometry-independent radionuclide value may be more
accurate.
Special attention must be paid to statistics with first pass ejection
fractions. Usually, the individual cardiac cycles in the first pass are
summed to produce a statistically reliable "super-beat" which may then be
displayed as a time-volume curve in the same way as in gated studies
(Thrall et al 1980). Other ways of improving the statistics from first
pass studies are by temporally smoothing the data (Dymond et al 1982b) or
by a root mean square procedure (Schelbert et al 1975). Large errors may
occur in ejection fractions due to low counts, and the clinical impact
of such errors may be enormous. For example, if the summmed background
counts in the left ventricle total only 500, then a true ejection
fraction of 40% could be represented as 30% or 50%, i.e. an error of 25%
merely due to poor statistics. Patients with ejection fractions of 50%
have a prognosis and operative survival which is superior to those of
patients with ejection fractions of 30%, and hence the decision making
process is ill-served by the potential for such errors. Similarly, if
intervention studies are performed, then an observed change in ejection
fraction from 50% to 30%, on the face of it a highly abnormal response,
could be due to errors based on poor statistics. With 5000 counts instead
of 500 the observed ejection fraction could range from 37% to 43%, an
error of only 8%. A constant review of count-rates provides a simple
method for continuing quality control in laboratories performing first
pass studies.
With proper attention to technical details, the radionuclide angiographic
ejection fraction is accurate, reproducible (Wackers et al 1979, Dymond
et al 1982b) and of major clinical value. It is important that each
laboratory establish its own normal and abnormal values at the inception
of a clinical programme.

6.Assessment of regional left ventricular function

The original method for assessing regional contraction patterns was to
outline the left ventricular contours at end-diastole and end-systole by
hand and to superimpose them, in the same way as for a contrast
angiogram. Akinesis was easily seen as points where the contours were
exactly superimposed. This approach has since been adapted for detecting
regional abnormalities using computer-generated ventricular outlines
(Marshall et al 1977, Dymond et al 1979, Thrall et al 1980). Although
clinically useful, there are important pitfalls in this method which are
related to the difficulty in detecting the exact ventricular edge. The
algorithms presently in use include isocount contours, or first or second
derivatives of profile curves across the left ventricle (Lieberman 1979).
The "wall motion image" may be inspected qualitatively or the degree of
inward motion measured using, for example, hemiaxial models (Stone et al
1980).
Wall motion may also be evaluated by inspection of the data in the
cinematic format. The entire gated study, or the first pass "super-beat"
may be shown on an endless loop as a representative cardiac cycle. In
this regard the cine differs from the contrast angiogram where individual
sequential beats are seen.
Neither contour images nor the cine display take full advantage of the
three-dimensional data present in a radionuclide angiogram. The contour
images in particular have the disadvantage of limited detection of
akinetic segments in regions that are not tangential to the detector

(Adam et al 1979). This has prompted the use of "functional" or
"parametric" imaging to exploit the three-dimensional information
present. Stroke volume images are formed by subtraction of the end-
systolic frame point by point .from the end-diastolic frame, and areas of
high stroke volume are depicted as areas of high intensity. The
superimposition of an end-diastolic contour aids appreciation of abnormal
anatomy (Thrall et al 1980). The regional ejection fraction image goes
one step further, by producing an image based on pixel-by-pixel time-
activity curves in the left ventricle. Regional contributions to ejection
fraction may be shown as different shades of grey or colour, and areas of
similar regional ejection fraction have the same shade or colour (Maddox
et al 1978, Dymond et al 1980). Calculation of regional ejection fraction
may also be effected by division of the end-systolic image into several
pie-shaped segments and calculating the ejection fraction of each
segment.
The most recent advance in functional imaging has been the development of
"phase images", which are constructed by using the first Fourier harmonic
to fit cosine curves to the time-activity curves of individual pixels
(Adam et al 1979). The cardiac cycle length may be divided into 360
degrees and the phase angle of each pixel is the angle at which the
cosine curve shows an initial decline. The behaviour of each element in
the cardiac image over the time course of a cardiac cycle is
characterised, and the resultant phase image allows visualisation of the
spatial distribution of differences in temporal behaviour. Thus, in the
normal heart, the atria and ventricles are 180 degrees out of phase, as
atrial contraction takes place during ventricular diastole and vice-
versa. Abnormal areas of wall motion within the ventricle are seen as
areas of abnormal phase, out of sequence with the normal myocardial
regions (Adam et al 1979). The use of these images to detect abnormal
sequence of ventricular activation will be discussed later. Phase images
have been mainly used with gated images where statistics are good; they
have not yet found wide application in first pass studies as statistics
in individual pixels are limited.

7.Calculation of ventricular volumes

As with ejection fraction, the earliest attempts to measure ventricular
volumes utilised the same area-length formulae which are applied to
contrast angiographic silhouettes (Strauss et al 1971) and this technique
has been widely applied. Reasonable correlations with contrast volumes
have been obtained even in patients with aneurysmal or myopathic hearts
(Dymond et al 1979). Nevertheless, the problems with edge detection have
made such measurements of limited value in intervention studies where
small changes in volumes need to be detected reproducibly and accurately,
and where small errors in edge placement will compound errors in volume
calculation. More recently, methods have been developed which allow
calculation of volumes from gated studies without resort to geometric
formulae, using the left ventricular activity related to blood activity,
converted to millilitres by regression analysis with contrast angiography
(Slutsky et al 1979a, Massie et al 1982). The count-density distribution
has also been used for non-geometric first pass volumes (Nickel et al
1982). Such measurements provide a lower standard error than geometric
values (Massie et al 1982).

8.Assessment of valvar regurgitation

The quantitative evaluation of left-sided valvar regurgitation requires
the simultaneous measurement of total and forward stroke volumes from
left ventricular cineangiograms and indicator dilution cardiac outputs,
regurgitant volume being the difference between the two. Rigo et al
(1979) introduced a new method for assessing valvar regurgitation using
the ratio of left ventricular to right ventricular stroke volume counts
from equilibrium gated images. In normal individuals, the stroke volume
from the two ventricles should be equal and the ratio should be unity. In
those with mitral and/or aortic regurgitation, the total stroke volume
from the left ventricle exceeds that of the right ventricle and the ratio
will increase. Janowitz and Fester (1982) showed that first pass studies
are also able to detect inter-ventricular differences in ejected stroke
counts in patients with valve regurgitation. Although the" regurgitant
index" has been subject to errors, particularly in patients with poor
left ventricular function or those with multiple extrasystoles (Lam et
al 1981),these techniques may be of value in patients where clinically
the degree of valve regurgitation is in doubt. This is particularly
likely to occur in the post-infarct patient or in those with prosthetic
cardiac valves, where the significance of cardiomegaly or murmurs is
uncertain. The method is not able to detect which valve is leaking (long
live the stethoscope!!) and of course is not applicable in the presence
of tricuspid regurgitation.

9.Phase analysis

The principles of phase imaging and its use in assessment of regional
contraction abnormalities have already been discussed. Currently, much
attention has been focussed on the ability of phase images to detect an
abnormal sequence of ventricular activation such as that occurring in
right or left bundle branch block (Frais et al 1982), or in ventricular
tachycardia (Swiryn et al 1982). Although this appears an expensive way
of diagnosing abnormalities which may be seen on electrocardiograms, the
consistency between electrophysiology and abnormal phase activation
provides some validation of the assumptions behind phase imaging. One
would anticipate that the major use of phase imaging in the future will
be to detect subtle abnormalities of right or left ventricular
contraction.

10.Right ventricular function

Radionuclide angiography has enabled the right ventricle to be studied
quantitatively in a manner similar to the left ventricle as the count-
volume relationship may be applied to this chamber equally. In fact,the
radionuclide techniques offer additional advantages over contrast
angiography, as the complex geometry of the right ventricle has precluded
the wide use of contrast studies for evaluation of right ventricular
function. The anatomical relationships of the right ventricle to the
right atrium and to the left side of the heart impose constraints on the
choice of projection for these studies. With equilibrium studies in the
left anterior oblique, there is substantial overlap between right atrium
and right ventricle throughout the cardiac cycle (Berger and Matthay
1981) and the contribution of right atrial counts to right ventricular
counts is difficult to overcome. The best separation between right atrium
and ventricle is achieved in the shallow right anterior oblique view,

which means that first pass techniques will be better suited to these studies. The lack of a suitable independent standard with which to compare radionuclide measurements of right ventricular ejection fraction has been a drawback, but several clinically useful applications of the information have already been made, especially in patients with chronic obstructive airways disease (Berger and Matthay 1981), and cystic fibrosis (Matthay et al 1980). The use in ischaemic heart disease is mainly to aid in the recognition of right ventricular infarction, which is particularly likely to occur in patients with inferior wall infarctions (Tobinick et al 1978).

11. Ejection and filling phase indices

In addition to left ventricular ejection fraction, these indices may be obtained from the time-volume curves of radionuclide angiograms. In 1976, Steele et al described the measurement of circumferential fibre shortening velocity from curves constructed over the minor axis of the ventricle. Marshall et al (1977) calculated normalised mean ejection rate by fitting a weighted least squares straight line to the systolic portion of the time-volume curve, and normalising the slope (dc/dt) to the average counts over the ejection phase. It was suggested that systolic ejection rate was a superior index of contractility to ejection fraction, as ejection rate increased with inotropic drugs whereas ejection fraction did not. One of the problems with this approach is that limited temporal resolution leads to a small number of data points in the systolic portion of the time-volume curve. Curve fitting techniques will be subject to errors if there are too few points on the curve. Thus, at a heart-rate of 60 beats per minute, and a framing rate of 20 per second, there will be 20 frames per cardiac cycle of which approximately half will be in the downslope. At 50 frames per second, there will be 50 frames per cycle. At heart-rates of 150 beats per minute, which may occur on exercise, 20 frames per second would only produce 8 frames per cycle, which is inadequate for curve fitting.

A great deal of interest has been shown in the early systolic portion of the time-volume curve, and in particular whether the "first third" ejection fraction is a more sensitive marker of impaired ventricular function than total ejection fraction. Slutsky et al (1979b) claimed that subtle abnormalities could be identified in patients with coronary disease using this measurement, but others have not found it useful (Kemper et al 1982). To date, the issue remains unresolved.

Assessment of diastolic function from the relaxation part of the time-volume curve has been described by Reduto et al (1981) from first pass studies, and by Bonow et al (1981) from gated studies. The interest in diastolic function stems from the fact that impairment of diastolic performance during ischaemia may occur even in the absence of systolic dysfunction. The effect of drugs on diastolic function may also be evaluated.

12. The non-imaging nuclear probe

A recently developed and increasingly popular alternative approach using the labelled blood-pool at equilibrium involves a non-imaging, portable scintillation probe. This instrument is sensitive enough to generate a real-time continuous left ventricular time-activity curve without resort

to ECG gating. Ventricular function may be assessed on a beat-to-beat
basis. Probe positioning is a crucial step if ejection fraction, relative
left ventricular volumes, and ejection and relaxation phase indices are
to be measured accurately. With practice in positioning, probe
measurements of ventricular function agree closely with those from
scintillation cameras (Berger et al 1981, Strashun et al 1981). The
advantages of this system are its low cost and portability, but the
disadvantage is that there are no images for the assessment of
ventricular size or of regional ventricular function which limits its
use as a primary diagnostic tool. The high temporal resolution (10 msec)
and high sensitivity make the system ideal for measurement of ejection
and relaxation phase indices.

13.Clinical role of radionuclide angiography

A complete discussion of the role that radionuclide angiography occupies
in the practice of clinical cardiology merits a text-book in its own
right, and the tables in the chapter by Elliott (these Proceedings)
outline the clinical uses briefly.
Resting studies are mainly used for a non-invasive quantification of
global and regional left ventricular function. The evaluation of
cardiomegaly, the detection of left ventricular aneurysms, the
differentiation between these and myopathic ventricles, and the
assessment of the extent of myocardial infarction, are all carried out to
decide whether left ventricular function is good enough for a patient
with severe cardiac failure, for example, to undergo cardiac surgery.
Where a discrete ventricular aneurysm is shown, then the next step may be
cardiac catheterisation. If there is severe diffuse impairment of
function, then catheterisation may not be advisable. The assessment of
patients receiving cardiotoxic drugs such as Adriamycin is important as
detection of early deterioration in ventricular function may allow the
drug to be stopped before a frank myopathy has developed (Alexander et al
1979). Nuclear angiography may be complementary to cardiac
catheterisation in cases where contrast angiography is not possible, or
be used for quantification of valvar regurgitation and evaluation of
intracardiac shunts. Finally, baseline studies provide the basis for
longitudinal follow-up studies to assess efficacy of therapy, e.g. in
patients with myocarditis receiving steroids.

The ability to study cardiac function under stress has made the exercise
radionuclide angiogram in many cases the raison d'etre of nuclear
cardiology. Patients with coronary artery disease may have entirely
normal left ventricular function at rest, but on exercise the ejection
fraction may fall and regional contraction abnormalities develop in
ischaemic areas. A large wealth of experience has now been gathered on
the behaviour of the normal and ischaemic ventricle under stress (Borer
et al 1979, Berger et al 1979, Stone et al 1980, Upton et al 1980,
Gibbons et al 1981, Slutsky 1981). There is little doubt that the
exercise radionuclide ventriculogram has improved the diagnostic
capabilities of exercise testing in coronary artery disease, as well as
the assessment of surgical treatment (Hellman et al 1980). Other clinical
uses of exercise studies include evaluation of drugs, and assessment of
functional reserve in patients with valve regurgitation which may aid in
the timing of surgical intervention. The technique allows regular non-
invasive follow-up of patients with known disease and permits appraisal
of the results of therapy.

Finally, other interventions may be of clinical use, e.g.
1) administration of nitroglycerine may improve function in asynergic segments and aid surgeons in the decision as to whether to by-pass a diseased coronary artery (Salel et al 1976).
2) the study of left ventricular function in patients being considered for programmable pacemakers may allow objective choice of the optimum mode of pacing for individual patients.

14.Conclusion

None of the aforementioned radionuclide techniques are perfect non-invasive tests of cardiac function. They are often expensive to establish in a hospital (although the tests themselves are cheap) and the limited spatial resolution means that delineation of cardiac anatomy will never be as good as with contrast angiography. The "trade-off" is the flexibility, ease of repetition and the ability to perform intervention studies. The technical requirements for dynamic cardiac imaging are many and careful attention to detail is mandatory if the results of radionuclide investigations are to be accepted by a still sceptical cardiological community. The physiological data available from nuclear imaging is complementary to the anatomical data obtained by other investigative techniques, and this can only lead to more complete patient care.

References

Adam WE, Tarkowska A, Bitter F, Stauch M and Geffers H 1979 Cardiac Nuclear Medicine (Berlin: Springer-Verlag)pp 21-33
Alexander J, Dainiak N, Berger HJ, Goldman L, Johnstone D, Reduto L, Duffy T, Schwarz P, Gottschalk A and Zaret B 1979 N.Engl.J.Med. 300 278
Berger HJ, Reduto LA, Johnstone DE, Borkowski H, Cohen LS, Langou RA, Gottschalk A and Zaret BL 1979 Am.J.Med. 66 13
Berger HJ and Matthay RA 1981 Am.J.Cardiol. 47 950
Berger HJ, Davies RA, Batsford WP, Hoffer PB, Gottschalk A and Zaret BL 1981 Circulation 63 133
Bonow RO, Leon MB, Rosing DR, Kent KM, Lipson LC, Bacharach SL, Green MV and Epstein SE 1981 Circulation 65 1337
Borer JS, Kent KM, Bacharach SL, Green MV, Rosing DR, Seides SF, Epstein SE and Johnston GS 1979 Circulation 60 57
Burow RD, Strauss HW, Singleton R, Pond M, Rehn T, Bailey IK, Griffith LC, Nickoloff E and Pitt B 1977 Circulation 56 1024
Cohn PF, Gorlin R, Cohn LH and Collins JJ 1974 Am.J.Cardiol. 34 136
Dymond DS, Jarritt PH, Britton KE and Spurrell RAJ 1979 Br.Heart J. 41 68
Dymond DS, Camm J, Stone D, Rees S, Rees G and Spurrell RAJ 1980 Br.Heart J. 43 270
Dymond DS, Elliott AT, Stone D, Hendrix G and Spurrell RAJ 1982a Circulation 65 311
Dymond DS, Halama J and Schmidt DH 1982b J.Nucl.Med. 23 1
Dymond DS, Elliott AT, Flatman W, Stone D, Bett R, Cuninghame G and Sims H 1983 J.Am.Coll.Cardiol.(in press)
Elliott AT, Dymond DS, Stone DL, Flatman W, Bett R, Cuninghame JG, Sims HE and Willis HH 1983 Phys.Med.Biol. 28 139

Flatman WD, Dymond DS, Dyke L, O'Keefe J and Short M 1983
Nuc.Med.Comm. (abstr) in press
Folland ED, Hamilton GW, Larson SM, Kennedy JW, Williams DL and
Ritchie JL 1977 J.Nucl.Med. 41. 1159
Frais MA, Botvinick EH, Shosa DW, O'Connell WJ, Scheinman MM, Hattner
RS and Morady F 1982 Am.J.Cardiol. 50 95
Gibbons RJ, Lee KL, Cobb F and Jones RH 1981 Circulation 64 952
Goris ML, Daspit SG, McLaughlin P and Kriss J 1976 J.Nucl.Med. 17
744
Hellman CK, Kamath ML, Schmidt DH, Anholm J, Blau F and Johnson
WD 1980 J.Thorac.Cardiovasc.Surg. 79 645
Janowitz WR and Fester A 1982 Am.J.Cardiol. 49 85
Jones RH, Sabiston DC, Bates BB, Morris JJ, Anderson PAW and Goodrich
JK 1972 Am.J.Cardiol. 30 855
Kemper AJ, Bianco JA, Shulman RM, Folland EF, Parisi AF and Tow DE
1982 Circulation 65 1094
Knapp WH, Dymond DS, Malfanti PL, Pachinger O, Sochor H, Vyska K and
Walton S 1981 Eur.Heart J. 2 97
Lam W, Pavel D, Byrom E, Sheikh A, Best D and Rosen K 1981
Am.J.Cardiol. 47 292
Lieberman DE 1979 Cardiovascular Nuclear Medicine (St. Louis: Mosby)
pp 76-102
Maddox DE, Holman BL, Wynne J, Idoine J, Parker JA, Uren R, Neill JM
and Cohn PF 1978 Am.J.Cardiol. 41 1230
Manyari DE, Nolewajka AJ, Purves P, Donner A and Kostuk WJ 1982
Circulation 65 571
Marshall RC, Berger HJ, Costin JC, Freedman GS, Wolberg J, Cohen LS,
Gottschalk A and Zaret BL 1977 Circulation 56 820
Massie BM, Kramer BL, Gertz EW and Henderson SG 1982 Circulation 65
725
Matthay RA, Berger HJ, Loke J, Dolan TF, Fagenholz SA, Gottschalk A
and Zaret BL 1980 Br.Heart J. 43 474
Nickel O, Schad N, Andrews J, Fleming JW and Mello M 1982 J.Nucl.Med.
23 404
Parker JA, Secker-Walker R, Hill R, Siegel B and Patchen EJ 1972
J.Nucl.Med. 13 649
Prinzmetal M, Corday E, Bergman HC, Schwarz L and Spritzler RJ 1948
Science 108 340
Reduto LA, Wickemeyer WJ, Young JB, Del Venturo LA, Reid JW, Glaeser
DH, Quinones MA and Miller RR 1981 Circulation 63 1228
Rigo P, Alderson PO, Robertson RM, Becker LC and Wagner HN 1979
Circulation 60 306
Salel AF, Berman DS, DeNardo GL and Mason DT 1976 Circulation 53
975
Schelbert HR, Verba JW, Johnston AD, Brock GW, Alazraki NP, Rose FJ
and Ashburn WL   1975 Circulation 51 902
Slutsky R, Karliner J, Ricci D, Kaiser R, Pfisterer M, Gordon D,
Peterson K and Ashburn W 1979a Circulation 60 556
Slutsky R, Gordon D, Karliner J, Battler A, Walaski S, Verba J,
Pfisterer M, Peterson K and Ashburn W   1979b Am.J.Cardiol. 44 459
Slutsky R 1981 Am.J.Cardiol. 47 357
Steele P, LeFree M and Kirch D 1976 Am.J.Cardiol. 37 388
Stone D, Dymond D, Elliott AT, Britton KE, Banim SO and Spurrell RAJ
1980 Br.Heart J. 44 208
Strashun A, Horowitz SF. Goldsmith SJ, Teicholz LE, Dicker A, Micel K
and Gorlin R 1981 Am.J.Cardiol. 47 610

StraussHW, Zaret BL, Hurley PJ, Natarajan TK and Pitt B 1971
Am.J.Cardiol. 28 575
Swiryn S, Pavel D, Byrom E, Bauernfeind RA, Strasberg B, Palileo E,
Lam W, Wyndham CRC and Rosen KM 1982 Am.Heart J. 103 319
Thrall JH, Pitt B and Brady TJ 1980 Nuclear Cardiology For Clinicians
New York: Futura) pp 165-186
Tobinick E, Schelbert HR, Henning H, LeWinter M, Taylor A, Ashburn
WL and Karliner JS 1978 Circulation 57 1078
Upton MT, Rerych SK, Newman GE, Port S, Cobb FR and Jones R 1980
Circulation 62 341.
Van Dyke D, Anger HO, Sullivan RW, Vetter WR, Yano Y and Parker HG
1972 J.Nucl.Med. 13 585
Wackers FJTh, Berger HJ, Johnstone DE, Goldman L, Reduto LA, Langou
RA, Gottschalk A and Zaret BL 1979 Am.J.Cardiol. 43 1159
Walton S, Donaldson EA, Rowlands DJ, Shields RA, Testa HJ and Wrigley
C 1980 Br.Heart J. 44 518
Wynne J, Holman BL, Mudge GH and Borow KM 1981 Am.J.Cardiol. (abstr)
47 444

Single Photon Emission Tomography

R A Shields & D N Taylor

Manchester Royal Infirmary & Walsgrave Hospital, Coventry

Abstract   The potential role of emission tomographic methods in
cardiology is considered and an assessment is made of how successful
they have been in solving problems posed by conventional planar cardiac
imaging.

Physical aspects of three methods are described: the multiple pinhole
technique, the rotating slant-hole, and the rotating gamma camera.
The limitations imposed by incomplete angle sampling are discussed,
and performance characteristics described for each system. These are
related in each case to data observed in clinical studies.

Results are discussed for static images of the myocardium and for time-
gated images of the ventricular blood pool. These indicate improvements over planar imaging, with the rotating slant-hole performing
better than the multiple pinhole, and a well designed rotating camera
system having the greatest potential for artefact-free tomographic
imaging.

1. Introduction

A conventional radionuclide imaging system applied to the study of the
heart produces two-dimensional images in which activities at different
depths within this three-dimensional organ are superimposed. There are
currently three areas of application of nuclear cardiology techniques for
which this drawback creates significant difficulties:

i)   The detection of coronary artery disease by stress thallium imaging.
This method has been widely adopted (using conventional 'planar' imaging
techniques) and the results of ten published studies indicate a mean
sensitivity of 80% and a mean specificity of 91% (Taylor 1980). These
figures restrict the usefulness of the technique. One major determinant
of failure to detect a perfusion defect is the presence of activity above
and below the lesion which may reduce the contrast of the lesion image to
below the limit of detectability.

ii)   The assessment of regional wall motion by gated blood pool imaging.
Although visualisation at equilibrium is preferable to first pass methods
from the point of view of demands on instrumentation, the assessment of
wall motion, particularly in the infero-basal segments of the left
ventricle, is impaired by right-ventricular overlap.

iii) The quantification of ventricular function by gated blood pool
imaging. Both global and regional measurements of ejection fraction are

notoriously sensitive to estimates of background, and the latter mainly comprises activity underlying or overlying the ventricular cavity.

During recent years, several approaches have been made towards the solution of this problem by the development of techniques for tomographic imaging: the visualisation of activity in a plane, or set of planes, through the volume of interest. One class of techniques exploits positron-emitting radionuclides and coincidence detector systems to detect pairs of annihilation gamma-ray photons, but in this paper we concentrate on the more readily-applicable techniques which rely on developments of existing imaging instrumentation in conjunction with established 'single-photon' gamma-ray emitting radionuclides.

2. Methods

The three methods most widely described and adopted are reviewed here. The first two are 'collimator techniques' in which a conventional gamma camera is equipped with a special collimator system in order to acquire views from a limited range of angles. The information is processed to produce estimates of distributions in planes essentially parallel to the camera face - approximately parallel to the long axis of the patient - and this approach is thus sometimes known as longitudinal tomography.

The third approach uses a rotating gamma-camera system to acquire projections of the distribution of activity over a full 360 degree range. The data may be reconstructed to form transverse axial sections.

In cardiology it is important to note that 'sectional' views ideally relate to the cardiac axes, rather than the long axis of the patient. Such re-orientation can be achieved by positioning of the camera in collimator techniques, and by the use of more sophisticated reconstruction algorithms on data from a rotating camera.

2.1 The Seven-Pinhole Collimator (7PH)

Fig. 1 shows the imaging geometry of the seven-pinhole collimator, first described by Vogel and colleagues (1978). Images are obtained simultaneously of seven independent projections using the central area and six sectors of the camera crystal. A clinical study must be preceded by flood field and point source measurements for calibration. A computer is used to correct and re-align the seven images ready for the reconstruction of sections by a method as described below.

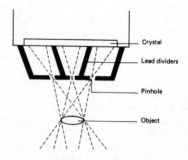

Fig. 1 Section through seven-pinhole collimator system.

2.2 The Rotating Slant-hole (RSH)

Fig. 2a indicates the basic geometry of the rotating slant-hole collimator system (Muehllehner 1971), in which the parallel holes of the collimator project a single image onto the crystal of a projection at a fixed angle, (typically 25°) to the normal. The collimator is rotated manually in 60° steps in order to acquire the angular samples in sequence.

A variation of this method, the quadrant slant-hole, is shown in Fig. 2b (Chang et al 1980). Four projections are acquired simultaneously, each using a quarter of the crystal area and thus covering a smaller field of view.

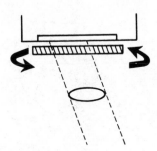

Fig. 2a Rotating slant-
hole collimator.

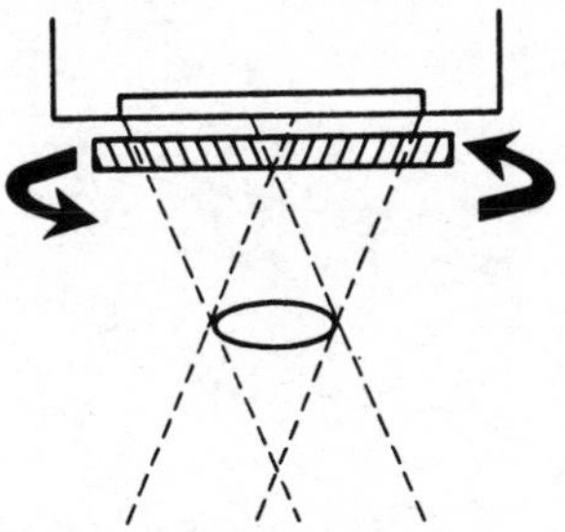

Fig. 2b Quadrant slant-
hole collimator.

2.3 Reconstruction of Sections (Collimator Methods)

The algorithms used to achieve the reconstruction are iterative solutions to the sets of simultaneous equations which define how the activities at corresponding points in sections of the object combine to form each projection image.   The success of this technique is dependent upon a good initial estimate of the sectional distribution; one approach is the use of an 'impedance operator' as illustrated in Fig. 3.   Three point sources of activity within the object volume (activities in the ratio 1:2:6) are shown projected onto three images.   The position within each image to which each source projects can be determined from the geometry.   The calculation shows how the value of an image pixel in any given plane can be estimated by forming the inverse of the sum of reciprocals of the total projected values.   In this simple example the three quantities emerge in their original ratios.   In practice we must deal with a continuous distribution of activity and

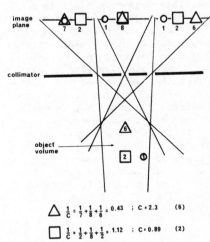

$$\triangle \quad \frac{1}{c} = \frac{1}{7} + \frac{1}{8} + \frac{1}{6} = 0.43 \quad ; \ C = 2.3 \quad (6)$$

$$\square \quad \frac{1}{c} = \frac{1}{2} + \frac{1}{8} + \frac{1}{2} = 1.12 \quad ; \ C = 0.89 \quad (2)$$

$$O \quad \frac{1}{c} = \frac{1}{7} + \frac{1}{1} + \frac{1}{1} = 2.14 \quad ; \ C = 0.47 \quad (1)$$

Fig. 3 The 'impedance operator' shown reconstructing the activities of three point sources in their original ratios.

each detected image element represents a line integral of the
distribution. The 'impedance operator' is used to give a first estimate
of the distribution in the set of planes, and the results are ray summed
to produce a new set of images. These are subtracted from the original
observed images to give a set of error images which are back-projected
(after relaxation) onto the reconstruction planes.

2.4 The Rotating Gamma Camera

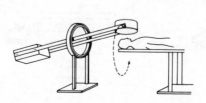 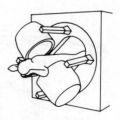

Fig. 4a Single-headed
rotating gamma camera.

Fig. 4b Dual-
headed rotating
gamma camera.

Fig. 4 indicates two designs of rotating gamma camera with which complete
sets of projection images may be acquired. Each line of a gamma-camera
image is a projection of a section of the distribution at a given angle.
The simplest method of reconstruction
is to back-project the recorded lines
onto an image plane, but as Fig. 5
shows, this does not result in a
faithful reproduction of the source.
The projections of a point source
back-project to give a star pattern.
An infinite number of projections
would back-project to give a falling-
off from the position of the point
as $1/r$, where r is the distance from
the point. The usual way to deal
with this is to convolve the
projection data with a spatial
operator before back-projection.
The operator is chosen such that
its effect is that of a ramp filter
in frequency space, rolled off to
supress the noise at high spatial
frequencies.

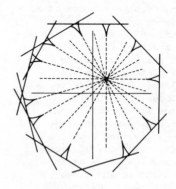

Fig. 5 Simple back-
projection of a point
source.

3. Results

3.1 The Seven-pinhole Collimator

The success of the technique in detecting perfusion defects will depend upon its ability to produce images of lesions with better contrast than planar imaging techniques. Fig. 6 shows the results of measurements on images of a phantom with a 3cm diameter lesion in successive tomographic cuts, indicated by plotting a contrast ratio which would ideally reach zero in the plane of the lesion and be unity outside the plane. In this example the conventional planar image, which does not of course discriminate in depth, detected the lesion with a contrast of 0.7. The tomographic cuts visualised the lesion with improved contrast in planes between 12 and 19cm in depth. Clinically this has been reflected in the higher sensitivity for detection of coronary artery disease and myocardial infarction reported in the literature.

In Table I we list the results of four studies which compared 7PH with planar images for detection of CAD. The mean sensitivity increased from 79% to 93% and specificity (the proportion of true negative results) remained approximately the same. A further three studies of detection of myocardial infarction however, show less encouraging results (Table II). The sensitivity of 7PH tomographic imaging is again improved over planar imaging (from 80% to 89%), but here the specificity is greatly reduced – from 91% to 70%. A likely explanation of the greater incidence of false positives is the presence of image artefacts.

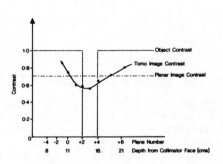

Fig. 6 Visualisation of a 3 cm diameter lesion at depth using a seven-pinhole collimator. (Williams et al 1980).

Reference	PLANAR IMAGING %		7-PINHOLE %	
	Sens.^{y}	Spec.^{y}	Sens.^{y}	Spec.^{y}
Vogel et al (1979)	74	96	95	96
Berman et al (1980)	87	90	91	90
Francisco et al (1980)	81	65	91	94
Rizi et al (1981)	75	91	94	91
Mean	79	86	93	93

TABLE I

SEVEN-PINHOLE TOMOGRAPHY FOR THE DETECTION OF CORONARY ARTERY DISEASE.

TABLE II

SEVEN-PINHOLE TOMOGRAPHY FOR THE DETECTION OF MYOCARDIAL INFARCTION.

Reference	PLANAR IMAGING		7-PINHOLE	
	Sens.^{y} %	Spec.^{y}	Sens.^{y} %	Spec.^{y}
Lewis et al (1981)	86		91	
Tamaki et al (1981)	75	89	93	68
Ritchie et al (1980)	80	93	83	71
Mean	80	91	89	70

3.2 The Rotating Slant-hole

The RSH system, like the 7PH system is capable of an image resolution of approximately 10mm FWHM at 10cm depth. However, the depth resolution (separation between resolvable planes) is maintained to greater depth by the RSH. Fig. 7 demonstrates this effect by plotting the observed depth resolution against depth for the two systems.

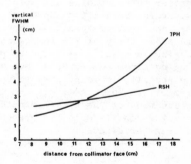

Fig. 7 Depth resolution of collimator systems.

Clinical experience to date with the RSH for stress thallium imaging does not, however, indicate a major improvement over planar studies. Again, there is some evidence that this may be due to the presence of artefacts influencing the incidence of false positive results. Studies at Coventry have demonstrated a non-uniformity of response in images of a ventricular myocardial phantom, dependent upon the orientation of the camera to the axis of the ventricle. Ratib et al (1982) have reported this observation and suggest an explanation based upon the partial volume effect, but doubts also exist about the accuracy of the reconstruction algorithms.

3.3 The Rotating Gamma Camera

Several implementations of rotating camera systems are now commercially available. The technique is capable of producing images of sections with resolutions of the order of 10mm FWHM and, in contrast to the collimator methods, the resolution and separation between resolvable planes do not deteriorate significantly with increasing depth (Flower et al 1981). For the successful development of this technique the following considerations are particularly important:

i)   The camera must have very good spatial linearity.

ii)   The linearity and uniformity should be independent of head orientation.

iii)   The rotation system must maintain a constant isocentre.

iv)   The reconstruction software should permit selection of orientation of the slices, so that these may be aligned with the major cardiac ventricular axes.

Table III summarises some early assessments of accuracy of these systems in detecting myocardial infarction with thallium imaging. They indicate an improvement in sensitivity with no loss of specificity.

TABLE III

ROTATING GAMMA CAMERA FOR THE DETECTION OF MYOCARDIAL INFARCTION.

Reference	PLANAR IMAGING Sens.^{y}% Spec.^{y}		ROTATING G.C. Sens.^{y}% Spec.^{y}	
Tamaki et al (1981)	75	89	96	89
Ritchie et al (1981)	61		100	
Maublant et al (1982)	89	93	98	93

It is possible to use the system for ventricular ejection studies by acquiring an ECG multiple time-gated sequence at each of the projections and subsequently sorting the data to produce multiple time-gated sequences in selected transverse sections (Shields 1982). From these data sectional volume curves and ejection fractions may be derived. The clinical significance of these results has yet to be assessed.

4.   Conclusions

Early seven-pinhole results indicate an improvement in sensitivity to perfusion defects, but this may be at the expense of specificity.

The rotating slant-hole system gives better separation of reconstruction planes, especially at some distance from the collimator. Results however are currently adversely affected by false positive defects caused by reconstruction artefacts. The rotating gamma camera, whilst a more complex system, is capable of better depth resolution than either collimator system and offers the greatest potential for an improvement in diagnostic accuracy.

References

Berman D S, Staniloff H, Freeman M et al 1980 Am. J. Cardiol. **45** 481

Chang W, Lin S L, Henkin R E 1980 Proc. Symp. Soc. Nucl. Med. Computer Council, Miami Beach, Florida pp 81-94

Flower M A, Rowe R W, Webb S et al 1981 Phys. Med. Biol. **26** pp671-691

Francisco D, Go R, Collins S et al 1980 Am. J. Cardiol. **45** 482

Lewis S E et al 1981 J. Nucl. Med. **22** 6 53

Maublant J, Cassagnes J, LeJeune J J et al 1982 J. Nucl. Med. **23** 204-208

Muehllehner G 1971 Phys. Med. Biol. **16** pp 87-96

Ratib O, Henze E, Hoffman E et al 1982 J. Nucl. Med. **23** pp 34-41

Ritchie J L, Caldwell J H, Williams D L 1980 Am. J. Cardiol. **45** pp 481

Rizi H R, Kline R C, Thrall J H 1981 J. Nucl. Med. **22** pp 493-499

Shields R A 1982 Measurement of ventricular ejection fraction using SPECT Proc. 3rd World Congress, WFNMB, Paris

Tamaki N, Mukai T, Ishii Y et al 1981 J. Nucl. Med. **22** pp 849-855

Taylor D N 1980 The assessment of the function and status of the left ventricle using radionuclides. Ph.D.Thesis (Univ. of Southampton)

Vogel R A, Kirch D, LeFree M et al 1978 J. Nucl.Med. **19** pp 648-654

Vogel R A, Kirch D L, LeFree M et al 1979 Am. J. Cardiol. **43** pp787-793

Williams D L, Ritchie J L, Harpe E D et al 1980 J. Nucl. Med. **21** pp 821-828

Short-Lived Radionuclides in Studies of Coronary Blood Flow and Myocardial Metabolism

M J Shea, R A Wilson, J I Deanfield, C M de Landsheere and A P Selwyn

MRC Cyclotron Unit and Cardiovascular Unit, Hammersmith Hospital, London, W12 OHS.

1. Introduction

The past decade has witnessed a revolution in new imaging techniques for cardiovascular investigation ranging from ultrasound to nuclear magnetic resonance and emission computed tomography. The most widely used techniques, ultrasound and contrast radiography, serve the clinician well in day-to-day patient management. From the investigative point of view, the new frontier will centre on physiologic studies of coronary blood flow and tissue metabolism. The attraction of PET is related to the union of its instrumentation with tracer theory providing the theoretical capability of quantitating physiologic processes in small tissue volumes, and the properties of positron-emitting radioisotopes which may be incorporated in a wide range of compounds from natural substrates and their analogues to drugs and antibodies.

2. Instrumentation and Positron Emission Tomography (PET)

The technique of PET depends on the unique collision of a positron with an electron resulting in annihilation photons of 511 KeV travelling in opposite directions. A scanner with multiple arrays of scintillation detectors surrounding this event will record and accept the event only if the two photons are detected simultaneously. Otherwise the information will be viewed as random events and therefore rejected. As the tissues between the positron-electron collisions and the detector may affect the passage of the two photons, transmission scans of tissue density are needed for attenuation correction. The detectors record each annihilation as a projection representing the pathway of the twin photons. The many projections arising from the annihilations in the tissue can be back-projected in a computer. The concentration and crossover of projections in different regions represent the concentration and distribution of tracer within the field of view. Algorithms are used to identify the structure and correction for tissue density is made so that the "emission scan" emerges as an image of a single slice of the heart, a "breadloafed" or tomographic slice that faithfully demonstrates the concentration of tracer in regions of myocardium.

The resolution of this technique is currently in the range of 8-15 mm, although scanners with a resolution of 2-3.5 mm are under construction (Muehllener & Colsher 1982). For heart studies, the current scanners are somewhat limited since the human heart wall is 0.6 - 1.2 mm thick. From the phantom studies of Hoffman and Phelps (1979), it appears that count recovery varies as a function of object size, i.e. the partial volume effect. For the heart, a 50% loss of counting efficiency can be expected unless appropriate recovery corrections are employed. The use of echocardiography to measure wall thickness has been used. If an intravascular scan (C - 11 carbon monoxide) is scaled and subtracted from transmission data, the extravascular myocardial density remaining may provide the appropriate correction factor.

Future improvements in instrumentation will involve not only spatial resolution but image quality as well. A new exciting generation of "time-of-flight" detectors are currently under construction. These machines will improve image quality by eliminating some of the uncertainty in timing of photon flight which contributes to positional uncertainty in event detection.

For further details on instrumentation, the reader may find several recent reviews helpful (Goodwin 1980, Ter-Pogossian 1981, Muehllener and Colsher 1982).

3.   Positron Emitting Radiopharmaceuticals

A major advantage of PET involves quantitation of physiologic processes because of the nature of positron-emitting radiopharmaceuticals.   The most frequently used positron-emitting radioisotopes and their half-lives are listed in Table 1.

The organic positron-emitters such as carbon-11 (C-11), nitrogen-13 (N-13) and oxygen-15 (O-15) can be incorporated into naturally occurring substrates without changing the organism's acceptance of these substrates as "the real thing", an issue of obvious importance for metabolic studies.

The most extensively studied radio-pharmaceutical for heart research is C-11 palmitate, a naturally occurring fatty acid.   Prior to the synthesis of palmitate (Klein et al 1979), fatty acids had been labelled with non-positron radionuclides in the w-position and concern has always lingered about possible biological interference by these radionuclides.

TABLE 1.   FREQUENTLY USED POSITRON-EMITTING RADIOISOTOPES

Radioisotope	Half-life (min)
Carbon-11	20.1
Nitrogen-13	10.0
Oxygen-15	2.1
Fluorine-18	109.0
Gallium-68	68.0
Rubidium-82	1.2

In certain situations biological interference may be advantageous.   For the study of carbohydrate metabolism the use of radiolabelled glucose was problematic because of its rapid metabolism.   An analogue, deoxyglucose, was found to be ideal for measuring glucose uptake as it was phosphorylated but was then metabolically trapped in the cell (Sokoloff et al 1977). Subsequent modifications, including the development of the fluorine-18 analogue (FDG), have allowed for the trapping of a positron-emitting molecule with a suitable residence time for positron tomography (Reivich et al 1977).

Given two different radioisotopes for labelling the same molecule, the differences in observed phenomena are best illustrated with recent investigations of amino acid metabolism. Henze et al (1982) examined N-13 and C-11 labelled amino acid kinetics during control and ischaemic conditions. Following myocardial uptake, N-13 amino acids underwent transamination with the N-13 label distributed to various amino acid pools.   The C-11 amino acids apparently entered the Krebs cycle and C-11 eventually appeared as $11\text{-}CO_2$.   Careful consideration of biochemical and patho-physiological aspects of a research problem followed by appropriate radioisotope selection may help avoid the unexpected or serendipitous result.

The choice of radioisotope may also depend on cost or convenience. Fluorine-18, because of its relatively long half-life, may be produced in one place (e.g. an institution with a cyclotron) but used in another (e.g. an institution without a cyclotron but with scanning capabilities). The vast majority of PET studies worldwide have used cyclotron-produced radio-isotopes for experimental and clinical studies. Rubidium-82, a generator produced potassium analogue, is used for serial studies of regional myocardial perfusion during myocardial ischaemia (Selwyn et al 1982b).Use of cyclotron-produced isotopes for such studies would be technically difficult and prohibitively expensive!

The ultimate choice of positron-emitting radiopharmaceutical depends on a blend of factors such as having a specific research question and need, identifying the measurements necessary to fulfil these needs, availability of cyclotron time, reliable tracer chemistry and the need to define units in a physiological model. With advancing improvements in radiochemical syntheses, and in particular the exciting developments in the labelling of membrane receptors and a variety of drugs, the only limitation to exploring these untapped areas may be the investigator's imagination.

4.   Positron Emission Tomographic Studies of the Heart

4.1 Measurement of Myocardial Blood Flow

Measurement of regional myocardial blood flow provides physiologic information which complements the anatomical information from the ventricular angiogram and coronary arteriogram. This information establishes a profile of ventricular health and defines the significance of coronary stenoses. The principle non-positron radionuclide techniques used to measure myocardial blood flow include xenon-133 administration into the coronary arteries (L'Abbate and Maseri 1980), krypton-81m administration also into the coronary arteries (Selwyn, and the popular clinical tool, thallium-201 scintigraphy (Pitt & Strauss, 1979) and the popular clinical tool, thallium-201 scintigraphy (Pitt and Strauss 1979). Each of these techniques has strength and drawbacks, recently reviewed by Allan and Selwyn (1982).
Quantitative measurements of blood flow per unit volume of myocardium have been attempted with several positron-emitting radionuclide agents including Ga-68 and C-11 labelled albumin microspheres, O-15 water, N-13 ammonia and rubidium-82. The positron labelled biodegradable albumin microspheres have great theoretical appeal as they represent a true flow marker. Injected into the left atrium of left ventricle, these micro-spheres are distributed to the heart and other organs in proportion to regional blood flows where they are trapped in capillary beds without recirculation. Wisenberg et al (1981) and Selwyn et al (1982a) demonstrated the utility of gallium-68 albumin microspheres as flow markers during experimental conditions of variable myocardial blood flows. The initial enthusiasm for this technique has tempered with recent information from our institution that the Ga-68 label may be disrupted by plasma components and leeched off with time. The long half-life of Ga-68 also makes it less desirable for human use because of the radiation dose to critical organs. Recently Turton (1983) and coworkers have developed a C-11 albumin microsphere which has ideal qualities: (a) stable heart

images are obtained with high myocardium to background ratios (> 10:1)
and no appreciable leeching of C-11 into the bloodstream (Fig.1) and (b)
regional myocardial blood flows determined with C-11 microspheres
correlate very well with a reference standard of blood flows determined by
long-lived gamma-emitting microspheres.   For human studies these microspheres will have the additional benefit of a radiation dose approximately
one-fifth that of the Ga-68 microspheres.   The human administration of
these microspheres will require catheterisation of the left ventricle, and
thus one can expect this technique to remain primarily a research
investigation for some time to come.

Positron Tomography : Experimental Studies

Cation Uptake   Myocardial Blood Flow

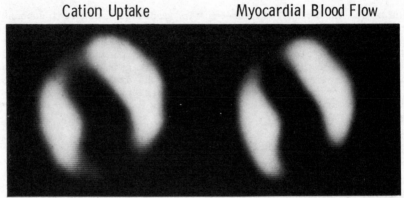

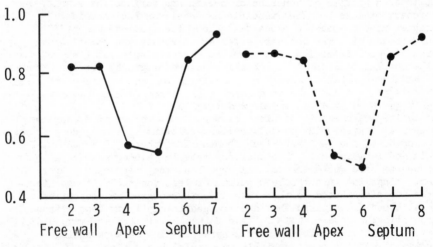

Fig.1   Positron tomographic studies of ischaemic canine myocardium.   The
left image demonstrates regional myocardial uptake of rubidium-82 (the
product of blood flow in ml/gm/min x extraction) with a graphic display
below.   The right image displays regional myocardial blood flow (ml/gm/
min) as determined by C-11 albumin microspheres.   Below this image is a
graphic display of flow in ml/gm/min.   Rubidium-82 uptake is directly
proportional to blood flow.

A method initially applied to brain studies utilises oxygen-15 water for measurement of regional myocardial blood flow (Allan et al 1981a). This technique is unique in that it requires the inhalation of short-lived radioactive gases, a completely noninvasive, safe and convenient approach for the patient. From Allan's preliminary studies it seems that there is a systematic relationship with perfusion at both low and high flows in the dog. In addition, studies in normal volunteers and patients suggested similar trends. In four patients with previous myocardial infarction, the infarcted regions demonstrated consistently decreased flow as compared to normal, noninfarcted regions. These studies utilised steady state techniques which are time consuming and difficult to employ for multiple scans in different physiological conditions. We are currently investigating bolus approaches to this problem.

An additional noninvasive approach to measurement of myocardial blood flow is that of intravenous injection of N-13 ammonia as described by Schelbert and coworkers (Schelbert et al 1979, 1981, 1982). In dog experiments they noted a rapid blood clearance of N-13 ammonia with a high extraction fraction of 72%. Myocardial tissue concentrations increased or decreased in relation to changes in flow although the changes were not truly linear, especially at high non-physiological flow rates. Bergmann and colleagues (1980) examined N-13 ammonia in an isolated rabbit heart model under varying conditions including hypoxia and during inhibition of glutamine synthetase, the enzyme likely to be responsible for the major metabolic trapping of NH_3. They found decreased uptake of N-13 ammonia with high flows, but with low flow there was not an increased uptake, presumably due to metabolic effects associated with low flow and hypoxia. With inhibition of glutamine synthetase, N-13 ammonia uptake was restricted while the heart preparation continued to function in an apparently normal fashion. Schelbert et al (1982) have studied normal volunteers and patients with coronary artery disease using N-13 ammonia at control conditions and after dipyridamole-induced hyperemia. From this work it appears that N-13 ammonia gives a directionally true indication of perfusion, however, in view of the experimental work of both Schelbert and Bergmann, it must be realised that N-13 ammonia does not act as an inert tracer. Instead, the determinants of its myocardial uptake are both blood flow and metabolic trapping, conditions which may have wide-ranging variability in ischaemic or unsteady states.

From the work of Yano et al (1979) and Horlock et al (1981) with subsequent modifications, we have seen the development of a generator producing the short-lived positron-emitting daughter of strontium-82, viz. rubidium-82. By eluting normal saline through the generator, rubidium-82 can be administered as an intravenous solution. The safety of the generator has been established: there is minimal breakthrough of strontium-82 and the sterility of the system can be maintained over 3-4 months despite multiple elutions for patient studies.

An intravenous infusion of rubidium-82 provides a steady-state in the patient's arterial blood within 2-3 minutes during which time a scan is performed. The infusion is then stopped and a "washout" scan is performed. By assigning a left ventricular region of interest to the steady-state scan, the arterial input function to the coronary arteries may be estimated and in turn division into the washout scan gives a measure of cation uptake. (The theoretical considerations of this technique have been discussed by Selwyn et al, 1982b). The short half-life of this agent allows for rapid steady-state formation, rapid cation

clearance and thus frequent scanning of transient event(s). This
technique makes a physiological measurement in each region of the
myocardial tomogram which is directly related to uptake (i.e. regional
myocardial flow, ml/gm/min x extraction of the tracer).

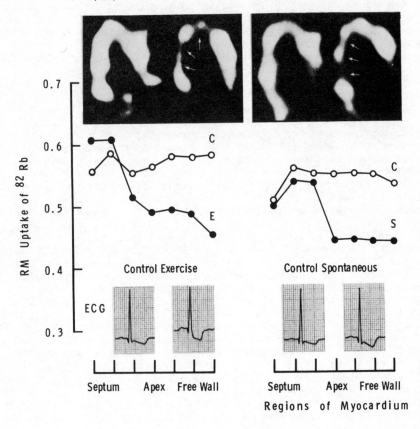

Fig.2   Rubidium-82 studies in a patient with ischaemic heart disease.
At rest,the rubidium uptake is uniform.   During exercise, the patient
developed angina pectoris and electrocardiographic signs of ischaemia.
The scan demonstrates an increased rubidium uptake in septal regions, the
normal response, whereas the apical and free wall regions have an
absolute decrease in uptake, an abnormal response.   A spontaneous
episode of ischaemia was heralded by a change in the electrocardiogram
while the patient was resting comfortably.   The free wall region
demonstrates an absolute reduction in cation uptake relative to the
normal control scan preceding this event.   Rubidium-82 is a reliable
marker of regional myocardial perfusion and is useful for serial studies
of ischaemic events of interest.

We have performed over 125 rubidium-82 positron tomographic studies in
patients with ischaemic heart disease.   Our typical patient has a normal
control or pre-intervention scan on first entering the scanner.   The
patients undergo supine bicycle exercise with increasing workloads until

angina pectoris or fatigue supervenes at which time the exercise is
stopped.   As with other interventions, careful note is made of the
patients symptoms, heart rate, blood pressure and electrocardiogram
before, during and after an intervention.   Serial scans during and
following exercise demonstrate abnormalities in the regional myocardial
uptake of rubidium-82:   "normal" areas increase cation uptake relative to
control scans while "abnormal" areas demonstrate either an absolute
decrease in cation uptake or a failure to increase cation uptake above
control values (Fig.2).   During recovery, angina disappears quickly while
the electrocardiogram takes somewhat longer to recover.   Of interest, we
have noted several patients have prolonged rubidium defects well beyond
the time of symptomatic and electrocardiographic recovery.   Whether this
prolonged recovery is a potential marker of prognosis or severity of
disease is unclear. Braunwald and Kloner(1982) have recently summarised
experimental work indicating that after an ischaemic insult the myocardium
may be "stunned" or "metabolically sick" for prolonged periods.   We are
pursuing both clinical and experimental studies to investigate this issue
further.   Of particular interest will be the assessment of the relative
contributions of disturbances of flow vs disturbances of metabolism during
the post-ischaemic recovery phase.   Preliminary clinical studies with
nitrates show a hastening of the prolonged recovery and "normalisation" of
rubidium uptake in abnormal regions.

After recovery, patients undergo a repeat exercise study or one of several
additional interventions.   From the repeated exercise studies, we have
found the regional perfusion defects to be highly reproducible within a
given study period as well as over periods of up to one year.

Additional "interventions" or "conditions" have included cold pressor
testing, isometric handgrip, hyperventilation, mental arithmetic, a large
meal, cigarette smoking or a drug intervention.   Regions of abnormal
rubidium uptake after such interventions tend to be the same as those
produced during exercise, although the uptake abnormalities are often
somewhat less severe.   In addition, the symptomatic, haemodynamic and
electrocardiographic responses may be quite variable suggesting that
different pathophysiological mechanisms may be at work at the onset of
transient ischaemia.

Of unusual interest, we have detected spontaneous episodes of impaired
regional perfusion in several patients undergoing evaluation with
rubidium-82 (Fig.2).   These episodes tend to be asymptomatic but are
often associated with ST segment depression.   Pari passu, 24-hour
ambulatory monitoring of the ST segment indicates frequent episodes of
asymptomatic ST depression in these patients suggesting that silent
myocardial ischaemia may be more common than previously appreciated
(Deanfield et al 1982).

Much like N-13 ammonia, rubidium-82 gives a reliable, directionally
correct index of perfusion, i.e. with low or absent cation uptake,
perfusion is diminished or absent.   This is of critical importance in
doing serial studies of ischaemic events.   The short-lived cation allows
repeatable studies using each patient as his own control.   This ability
to follow the symptomatic and asymptomatic episodes of transient
ischaemia is of fundamental importance to understand the pathophysiological events that complicate coronary atherosclerosis.   It
should be noted, however, that experimental work in the dog demonstrates

that rubidium uptake is dependent on both flow and metabolism Selwyn et al 1982b). We have extended these studies and shown that for any given animal, rubidium-82 uptake has a direct but individual relationship with flow as measured with C-11 albumin microspheres.

Rubidium-82 is a useful imaging agent which has two major advantages over most positron-emitting indicators of blood flow; (a) capability of repeated scanning at short intervals and (b) non-dependence on the cyclotron for its daily use. This latter feature is particularly valuable in allowing for flexibility in patient scheduling. The major disadvantage in the use of an agent such as this with such a short half-life is the potential to miss the ischaemic region. This problem is of greater importance when a single slice scanner is used. With slice level adjustment or, in some cases, repeated studies at different sittings, the missed ischaemia problem can be overcome.

4.2 Assessment of Regional Myocardial Metabolism

Early explanations of myocardial metabolism with positron tomography have been necessarily limited to answer two questions. Does the radiolabel give an adequate image of the heart? Does the radiolabel trace the event of interest? More recent studies have attempted to define the important issues of tracer/substrate physiology under varying conditions.

Long-chain fatty acids are the major source of energy for the heart under aerobic conditions (Rothlin and Bing 1961, Neely et al 1972). The long-chain fatty acid C-11 palmitate has been extensively evaluated as a tracer of fatty acid metabolism. Preparatory experimental studies demonstrated that C-11 palmitate uptake was qualitatively decreased during ischaemia (Weiss et at 1976). Subsequently, this agent proved useful for quantitative infarct sizing (Weiss et al 1977, Ter-Pogossian et al 1980, Geltman et al 1982). Elegant studies of C-11 palmitate kinetics by Schon and coworkers (1982a, b) have shown that the uptake of palmitate is similar in normal and ischaemic myocardium although the fate or clearance of this fatty acid is altered by ischaemia. They delineated three phases of disposition, vascular, early rapid and late slow phases. The vascular phase represents the movement of tracer through the vascular space. The early rapid phase is though to reflect beta-oxidation (as measured by $11\text{-}CO_2$ production) and is significantly smaller during ischaemia than in normal myocardium, presumably owing to the diversion of palmitate from oxidation to triglyceride formation. The late slow phase is least well understood but is felt to correspond to the slow turnover of esterified palmitate. As might be expected, this phase was larger during ischaemia, again due to the presumed shunting of the palmitate to triglyceride. This experimental work supports the concept that palmitate oxidation rates might be quantitatively measured using positron tomography.

Because of the oxidation of fatty acids like palmitate, an additional approach to investigating fatty acid metabolism has involved the design of a labelled fatty acid analogue which is minimally metabolised yet metabolically trapped in the myocardium. Livni and coworkers (1982) have synthesised beta methyl (1 C-11) heptadecanoic acid and demonstrated its potential usefulness as a myocardial tracer. In preliminary studies we have verified the efficacy of this agent in labelling canine myocardium with an excellent target to background ratio and stable images with essentially no biological degradation over 60 minutes.

Attempts at labelling short-chain fatty acids for myocardial imaging have generally been unrewarding.   Using C-11 pentanoate in the canine, we found persistent blood pool images of this tracer but very poor myocardial uptake.

Myocardial Clearance of 11 C -Acetate

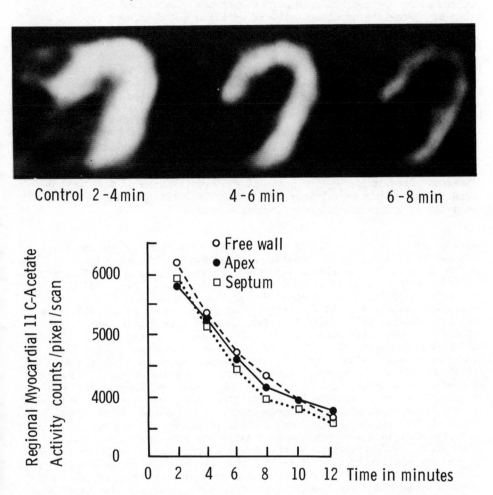

Fig.3   Myocardial clearance of C-11 acetate in a normal volunteer. The first image demonstrates a very "hot" myocardium with slight blood pool activity.   The second scan demonstrates uniform regional myocardial uptake of C-11 acetate with no blood pool activity.   The third scan (and subsequent scans not shown) demonstrates persistent homogenous C-11 acetate activity despite ongoing physical decay of the tracer.   In patients with ischaemia, C-11 acetate clearance is delayed from the ischaemic region.   Clearance studies may be useful in the positive labelling of ischaemic myocardium in addition to studies of Krebs cycle metabolism during various pathophysiological states.

The shortest chain fatty acid, acetate, labelled with C-11 is an effective tracer for myocardial imaging, although its theoretical appeal lies in its potential for investigating Krebs cycle activity as opposed to fatty acid metabolism.   In normal volunteers there is a uniform myocardial uptake of C-11 acetate following intravenous injection (Fig.3). The regional clearance of this tracer can be measured from scans of a single plane or from multiple planes when the question of ischaemia arises.   From the experimental work of Allan and coworkers (1981b) it appears that C-11 acetate has an early rapid phase of clearance somewhat similar to palmitate.   This unexpected finding raises more questions than it answers as the metabolism of acetate and palmitate presumably reflect different states, Krebs cycle activity in the former case and transport, beta-oxidation and Krebs cycle in the latter case.   Further investigations will be necessary to explain this finding.   Of equal interest is the observation that C-11 acetate clearance from ischaemic myocardium is significantly delayed in both an experimental canine preparation and man during transient ischaemia (Allan et al 1981b, Selwyn et al 1981).This delay in washout allows for a positive labelling of ischaemic areas which can be followed with serial scanning.   Clinical studies of C-11 acetate injected at the peaks of exercise identified ischaemic myocardium 10-15 minutes after normalisation of the electro-cardiogram.   Thus acetate may be a useful tool for studying Krebs cycle activity during prolonged post-ischaemic recovery.

Whereas fatty acids are the major metabolic substrate of the normal, aerobic myocardium, under conditions of ischaemia with anaerobic metabolism, glucose uptake is increased for energy production (Neely et al 1972).   Early studies of glucose metabolism in the rat brain led to subsequent modifications of experimental tracer kinetic models for the heart (Gallagher et al 1977, Phelps et al 1987, Ratib et al 1982).   Ratib and colleagues (1982), measuring tissue kinetics of FDG in the dog, showed the myocardial metabloic rate of glucose as judged by PET to be in good agreement with values obtained by direct arterio-venous sampling techniques over a wide range of glucose metabolic rates.   Schelbert et al (1982) extended this work in examining FDG uptake during experimental demand-induced ischaemia.   In ischaemic regions blood flow was reduced (measured with N-13 ammonia) while the FDG uptake was in excess of flow, a PET confirmation of basic experimental work.   Marshall et al (1981) found similar results in clinical studies of normal volunteers, patients with unstable angina pectoris and patients who were post-myocardial infarction.   In the normals as well as those post-infarction, the uptake of FDG was similar to that of N-13 ammonia and glucose uptake paralleled blood flow.   In patients with unstable angina with evidence of ongoing ischaemia,the FDG uptake was in excess of flow.   This was also true for a small group of patients with evolving myocardial infarction.   These exciting findings may be of use in future studies attempting to detect and salvage ischaemic myocardium at risk of infarction.

The measurement of glucose uptake seems possible using PET but there are some unanswered questions, e.g. are the lump constants and assumptions inherent in Sokoloff's equations valid for the derivation of glucose utilisation.   What are the separate effects of flow, capillary permeability and glucose transport?   These are issues under active investigation.

One of the more complex areas of current metabolic investigation centres on the fate of labelled amino acids.   These difficulties are related to the low affinity of myocardium for some amino acids with consequent appreciable recirculation, and the inherent complexities of intermediary metabolism.   Amino acids are delivered by blood flow, transported with energy consumed, variably shunted to a random pool, deaminated, oxidated and eventually incorporated into protein synthesis.   Any model for use with PET will have to "experiment out" these separate contributions. Gelbard et al (1980) injected N-13 glutamate into both normal volunteers and cancer patients but were only able to demonstrate a 5.7% myocardial uptake of the injected dose.   Henze et al (1982) explored a variety of amino acids labelled with either N-13 or C-11.   During experimental low flow ischaemia, the washout of N-13 amino acids was prolonged suggesting a possible "positive" label for ischaemic tissue.   The C-11 amino acids apparently entered the Krebs cycle as $11\text{-}CO_2$ was generated shortly after injection.   As with acetate, the C-11 amino acids may be useful in future studies of the Krebs cycle in various physiological states.   While there is obvious interest in studying the fates of these tracers during ischaemia, their potential value may be even greater in clinical disorders of the heart with known or suspected abnormalities of protein synthesis such as ventricular hypertrophy, cardiomyopathies and heart failure.

5.   The Future

The future of positron emission tomography depends on several inter-related issues: (a) clear clinical research questions regarding the mechanisms causing the diseases under study, (b) progress in instrument-ation with increased sensitivity and resolution during detection, (c) reliable radiochemistry and kinetic modelling that is relevant to the unit measurements required to address the questions in (a), and (d) physiological validation of the tracer and unit measurements to understand limitations followed by structured studies in well-characterised patients manifesting the disease under study.   All of these assumptions require the solid underpinnings of "biological information from basic science research as a prelude to clinical utility", to paraphrase Brownell et al (1982). From advances in these areas there can be no doubt that PET will contribute in a major way to the understanding of physiological processes in the normal and diseased heart.

Acknowledgments

We thank Pat Tierney for assistance in preparing this manuscript.

M.J.Shea is a Clinician-Scientist Awardee of the American Heart Association.   R.A.Wilson is a British-American Heart Fellow and Fulbright Fellow.   J.E.Deanfield is a Medical Research Council Fellow. C.M. de Landsheere is a NATO Fellow.

References

Allan R M, Jones T, Rhodes C J, et al 1981a Am J Card 47 481
Allan R M, Pike V W, Maseri A and Selwyn A P 1981b Eur J Card 2 A138
Allan R M and Selwyn A P 1982 Blood Flow Measurement in Man
   ed R T T Mathie (London:Castle) pp 83-98
Bergmann S R, Hack S, Tewson T, Welch M J and Sobel B E 1980 Circ 61 34
Braunwald E and Kloner R A 1982 Circ 66 1146

Brownell G L, Budinger T F, Lauterbur P C and McGeer P L 1982 Science 215
    619
Deanfield J, Fox K, Ribeiro P, et al 1982 Circ 66 II 17
Gallagher B M, Ansari A, Atkins H, et al 1977 J Nucl Med 18 990
Gelbard A S, Benna R S, Reiman R E, et al 1980 J Nucl Med 21 988
Geltman E M, Biello D, Welch M J, et al 1982 Circ 65 747
Goodwin P N, 1980 Sem Nucl Med 10 322
Henze, E, Schelbert H R, Barrio J R, et al 1982 J Nucl Med 23 671
Hoffman E J and Phelps M E 1979 J Comp Assist Tomog 3 299
Horlock P, Clark J, O'Brien H A, Grant P E and Bentley A 1981 J Radioanal
    Chem 64 257
Klein M S, Goldstein R A, Welch M J and Sobel B E 1979 Am J Physiol 237 H51
L'Abbate A and Maseri A 1980 Sem Nucl Med 10 2
Livni E, Elmaleh D R, Levy S, Brownell G L and Strauss W H 1982 J Nucl
    Med 23 169
Marshall R C, Schelbert H R, Phelps M E, et al 1981 Am J Cardiol 47 481
Muehllener G and Colsher J G 1982 Computed Emission Tomography eds P J
    Ell and B L Holman (Oxford) pp 3-41
Neely J R, Rovetto M J and Oram J F 1972 Prog Cardiov Dis 15 289
Phelps M E, Hoffman E J, Selin C, et al 1978 J Nucl Med 19 1311
Pitt B and Strauss H W 1979 Cardiovascular Nuclear Medicine eds
    H W Strauss and B Pitt (London:Mosby) pp 243-254
Ratib O, Phelps M E, Huang S C, et al 1982 J Nucl Med 23 577
Reivich M, Kuhl D, Wolf A, et al 1977 Acta Neural Scand 56 Supp 64 192
Rothlin M E and Bing R J 1961 J Clin Invest 40 1380
Schelbert H R, Phelps M E, Hoffman E J, et al 1979 Am J Cardiol 43 209
Schelbert H R, Phelps M E, Huang S C, et al 1981 Circ 63 1259
Schelbert H R, Henze E, Phelps M E and Kuhl D E 1982 Am Heart J 103 588
Schon H R, Schelbert H R, Robinson G, et al 1982a Am Heart J 103 532
Schon H R, Schelbert H R, Najafi A, et al 1982b Am Heart J 103 548
Selwyn A P, Steiner R, Kivisaari A, Fox K and Forse G 1979 Am J Cardiol
    43 547
Selwyn A P, Allan R M, Pike V, Fox K and Maseri A 1981 Am J Cardiol 47 481
Selwyn A P, Allan R M and Brady F 1982a Clin Sci 62 3
Selwyn A P, Allan R M, L'Abbate A, et al 1982b Am J Cardiol 50 112
Sokoloff L, Reivich M, Kennedy C, et al 1977 J Neurochem 28 897
Ter-Pogossian M M, Klein M S, Markham J, Roberts R and Sobel B E 1980
    Circ 61 242
Ter-Pogossian M M 1981 Sem Nucl Med 11 13
Turton D, Brady F, Pike V, et al 1983 Submitted for publication
Weiss E S, Hoffman E J, Phelps M E, et al 1976 Circ Res 39 24
Weiss E S, Ahmed S A, Welch M J, et al 1977 Circ 55 66
Wisenberg G, Schelbert H R, Hoffman E J, et al 1981 Circ 63 1248
Yano Y, Budinger T, Chang G, O'Brien H, Grant P 1979 J Nucl Med 20 961

Parametric Imaging of the Heart

N J G Brown, P H Jarritt and A S Houston.

Institute of Nuclear Medicine, The Middlesex Hospital Medical School, London W1, and R N Hospital, Gosport, Hants.

1. Introduction

By uclear cardiological techniques it is possible to obtain a set of digital images (frames) showing the distribution of counts from the heart at a set of equally spaced time intervals following the E.C.G. 'R' wave. Typically there will be sixteen frames each made up of 1024 count values arranged in an array having 32 columns and 32 rows. This data may be displayed as a set of static images or as a continuous cine cycle (movie mode). The quantitative information about the changing patterns of count-rate is not fully accessible from either of these forms of display. Furthermore the movie display cannot be put in the patient's notes! These problems can be overcome by the use of Parametric images designed to display quantitative information regarding specific aspects of the patterns of count rate variation throughout the cycle.

2. Parametric Images

The data making up the set of images may be arranged in a different way (Figure 1). If the first value in each image is taken in turn then a 16-point curve is obtained. This shows the variation in count-rate exhibited by the first pixel of the image during the cycle. This can be done for each pixel and so 1024 curves are obtained. These are referred to as individual pixel volume curves since the count-rate associated with a given pixel approximates the volume of blood present at the corresponding region in the patient. Quantitative information concerning some aspect of the pattern of volume change contained in an individual volume curve may be obtained by calculating some suitable function, such as the difference between the maximum and minimum values for example. If this calculation is performed for each of the 1024 curves and the different values obtained stored at the corresponding points of a 32 by 32 array, then the latter may be referred to as a difference parametric

image. Such an array of data can be readily displayed
by a Nuclear Medicine Computer system using the
routines originally provided to display the data
contained in count-rate digital images. When displayed
it demonstrates the regional variation in the
difference in count-rate (volume) between End-Diastole
and End-Sytole.

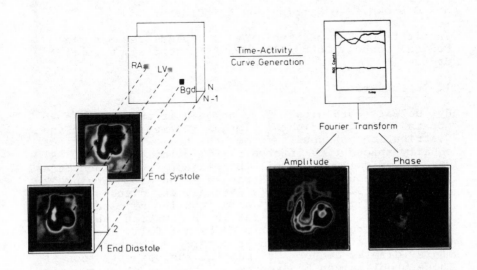

Fig 1 A set of equilibrium data may be looked at
in different ways.

The difference image has other uses. If an isocount
contour of about 20% of the maximum difference value
is displayed, this will be found to contain most
structures of interest which are beating. This contour
is often used to mask out regions of no significance in
other parametric images.

If the difference for each pixel is expressed as a
fraction of the maximum value for that pixel then a
parametric image showing the variation in the
fractional difference in count-rate is obtained. This
is generally referred to as the Regional Ejection
Fraction Image (REFI). Examples of these images are
shown in Figure 2. The image showing count-rate
difference is commonly called the amplitude image for a
reason which will be explained below. It may be noted
that the fractional difference image (REFI) has
comparatively greater values around the edge of the
ventricle where the count-rate falls to zero at End-
Systole as a result of wall motion, provided background
has been subtracted.

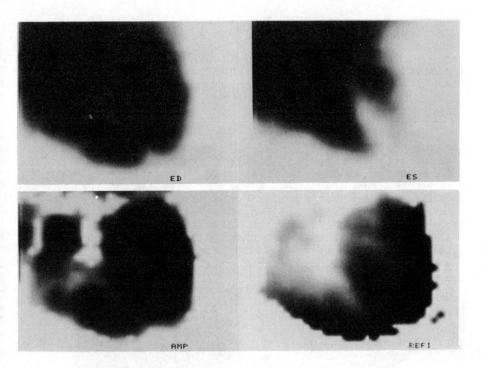

Fig 2   End-Diastolic (ED), End-Systolic (ES)
        frames and Parametric images.

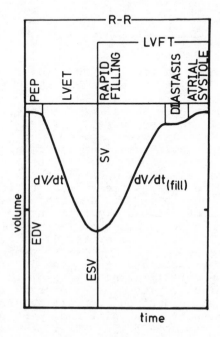

Fig 3 Some
quantities
obtainable
from the
volume curve

Some commonly measured quantities obtainable from the
volume curve are shown in Figure 3. In principle any of
these can be used to obtain a functional image provided
an adequate number of frames has been acquired. An
example of this is the ·peak ejection rate (Bacharach et
al 1980).

3. Time Images

So far we have only considered functions related to the
count — rate axis of Figure 3. However, the times at
which certain features of the curve occur are also of
interest. We can readily produce parametric images
showing the distribution of the timing of certain
events. These can be displayed in the same way as the
count based images. The most important times of
interest are the times of maximum and minimum count.
The images obtained from these time distributions have
been termed the time of End-Diastole (TED) and the time
of End-Systole (TES) respectively (Brown et al 1980).

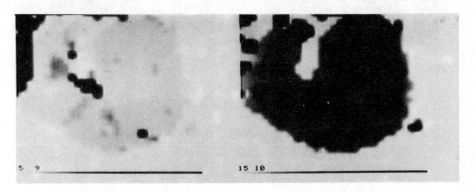

Fig 4   On the left TED (low frame values)
        on the right TES (higher values)

Examples are shown in Figure 4, taken from the same
normal case as Figure 2. These images were obtained by
simply identifying for each pixel the numbers of the
frames showing maximum and minimum count — rate. Thus
each point in the images can take on one of sixteen
values if, for example 16 frames of data were acquired.
With the grey scale representation of Figure 4, it is
only possible to see that there is a uniform
distribution of early frame numbers for the time of End
Diastole and a somewhat more varied variation of later
times for the time of End-Systole. If these images are
displayed using a colour scale consisting of 16
discrete colours, then the information regarding the
timings at different points of the image is transmitted
unambiguously to the observer. The TES image may be
refined if desired by fitting some function such as a
Gaussian to the point near the minimum of a curve in
order to obtain the time values to an accuracy

better than one frame. This needs to be displayed using a
continuous colour scale and the precise information
about timings is lost. However, there may well be
situations where information about small differences in
timings is more important than knowing absolute
timings.

A number of time images can be obtained from the data.
The most potentially useful, apart from TED and TES,
are probably the time of maximum rate of emptying and
the time of maximum rate of filling images.

4. The Phase Image

The most widely used time image at present is the
so-called Fourier Phase Image (Geffers et al 197).
These workers were the first to obtain parametric
images based on the coefficients obtained from the
Fourier series of the volume curves corresponding to
each pixel. They used only the first harmonic in their
Fourier series thus constraining the volume curve to
the form:

$$f(x) = k + a.\cos(x) + b.\sin(x) \quad \ldots\ldots\ldots\ldots 1$$

The first harmonic is characterised by two parameters
based on the coefficients a and b, these are the phase,
which is the angle whose tangent is given by b/a and
the amplitude, which is given by the square root of the
sum of the squares of a and b. They thus obtained phase
and amplitude images, examples of which for a normal
subject are shown in Figure 1. The amplitude image is
virtually identical to the difference image (hence the
usual name) since the amplitude reflects the maximum
excursions of the summed sine and cosine terms. The
clinical significance of the angle whose tangent is
given by b/a is not obvious, and there is no concensus
as to the implication of differences in phase value.
However, there is no doubt that the image clearly shows
the location of the ventricles and has greatly assisted
the reproducible definition of ventricular regions of
interest. Furthermore, gross differences in phase are
obtained in the case of aneurysms for example (Walton
et al 1981).

How does the phase vary with the shape of the curve?
The obscurity surrounding this question is dispelled
when the alternative form of the Fourier series is
used. It may be shown that:

$$a.\cos(x) + b.\sin(x) = c.\cos(x - \phi) \quad \ldots\ldots\ldots\ldots 2$$

where c is a constant determining the amplitude and ϕ
is the phase shift. It is clear from this that when
the first harmonic only is concerned the so -called
Fourier series is in fact simply the fit of a single

sinusoid to the volume curve. The amplitude and phase
(or shift along the time axis) being adjusted so as to
obtain the best fit between the sinusoid and the
observed curve. The constant k in equation 1 shifts
the sinusoid by an appropriate amount in the count
direction. It seems not unreasonable that this
sinusoid will roughly fit the gross feature of the
curve which is of course a trough for ventricular
pixels or a peak for atrial pixels.
Therefore the phase is a value which reflects in some
not very precise way the location of the entire curve.
By contrast, the time of End - Systole identifies a
specific time. It is open to question which of these
is likely to be the more clinically useful parameter.

5. Principle Components

Another approach which concerns a fit to the whole
curve, but which does not have the problem of
constraining the curve to a particular form, is that of
Principle Components analysis (also known as factor
analysis). This mathematical technique extracts the
fundamental components from which the 1024 curves of a
given study are made up (Houston et al 1982). A
polar transformation is required to obtain the
equivallent of phase and amplitude images. These have
the advantage that approximately the same value of
"phase" is obtained for all regions of normal ventricle
from patient to patient.

6. Conclusion

A large number of parametric images may be calculated.
They make use of the power of the modern computer to
demonstrate detail in a complex set of image data which
cannot be quantified by any other means. They are
valuable for transmitting complex information in an
unambiguous way.

References

Bacharach S L, Green M V, Borer S J, Hyde J E,
Farkas S P and Johnson G S 1979 J. Nucl. Med. 20 pp 189-
193
Brown N J G, Jarritt P H, Walton and Ell P J 1980 Nucl.
Med. Comm. 1 163
Geffers H, Adam W E and Bitter F 1978 Proc. Conf. Inf
Processing in Med. Imaging. ORNL/BICTIC pp 322-332
Houston A S, Elliott A T and Stone D L 1982 Phys. Med.
Biol. 27 pp 1269-1277
Walton S, Jarritt P H, Brown N J G, Ell P J and
Swanton R H 1981 B.M.J. 45 pp 348-350

Edge Detection and Wall Motion: An Intercomparison of Different Algorithms in Nuclear Cardiology

A. Todd-Pokropek
Department of Medical Physics, University College London, London, U.K.

1. Introduction: The aim of the study.

The aim of the study described here was to test various algorithms designed to determine the edge of the left ventricle, using both clinical and phantom material in Nuclear Cardiology. The imaging procedures used in Nuclear Cardiology, discussed at length elsewhere, will not be presented here. There is however a major problem: how can such algorithms be validated? This cannot be isolated from the question: what is the precise reason for trying to identify the left ventricle (LV)?

It could be as part of a procedure for:-

1. Determination of ejection fraction (EF)

2. Determination of a region within which various regional parameters such as regional EF might be determined

3. Determination of cardiac wall motion

For the purposes of this study, the main aim of such algorithms is considered to be primarily the first, partially the second, and not the third. Wall motion detection will be considered separately. It must be pointed out that similar algorithms are used in digital (cardiac) radiology, and similar procedures for testing them are required.

2. Types of algorithms

While various manual and totally automatic (and hybrid) algorithms have been described, this study was orientated to look at purely automatic algorithms since there is a strong suggestion that such algorithms can significantly improve reproducibility (Goris 1980) if not accuracy. Following the literature, algorithms looking at 'slope' in an image were initially considered, being specifically techniques to extract gradient and second differential. The phase image (or one of its variants such as the cosine image) as described by Geffers et al (1977) and Bossuyt et al (1980), may also be of considerable value in outlining the LV and will be considered later. However, the conventional isocount contour was discarded at an early stage since definition of the interventricular septum by this method seemed impossible.

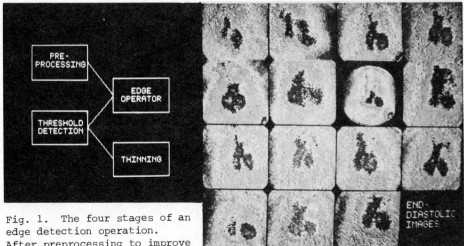

Fig. 1. The four stages of an
edge detection operation.
After preprocessing to improve
the signal-to-noise ratio, edge
detection must be followed by
a threshold operator and
thinning to produce a 'line'.

Fig. 2. A set of 15 consecutive end-
diastolic images, used as a test set.

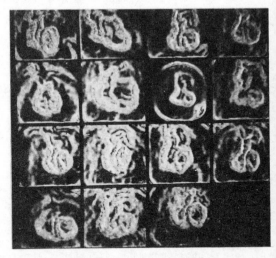

Fig. 3. The result of applying the
Wechsler edge operator to each of the
images shown in Fig. 2 above.

It should be stressed that these methods are not by any means exclusive and that, while the use of binary (Crisp) regions of interest (ROIs) is well ingrained into the manner of treating such studies, there exists a well developed formalism for fuzzy sets as presented by Zadeh (1970). Here instead, a pixel has a degree of belonging to one of the sets in the image (LV RV etc) combining several different measures of affinity for the pixel with respect to the set. One attribute for LV membership of particular interest is that of NOT RV, or its lack of affinity to the set of Right Ventricular pixels. In any case, at some point, a Crisp set has to be generated from the fuzzy set by use of a suitable thresholding operator. The use of phase information in this context will be considered later.

Following the literature (Rosenfeld et al 1971, Cahill et al 1976, Pratt 1978, Levialdi 1980) the following operators were considered:

1. Robert's gradient operator
2. Sobel gradient operator
3. Prewitt gradient operator
4. Kirsch gradient operator
5. Wechsler gradient operator
6. Template operators of the above types
7. Compass gradient operators of the above types
8. Ratio of variance operator
9. Nearest neighbour operator
10. Laplacian 2nd differential operators of different sizes

Note that the use of all such operators falls into four stages as illustrated in Fig. 1. There is:

Firstly, a preprocessing stage where a (preferably edge preserving) smoothing operation is employed to improve the signal-to-noise ratio in the image.

Secondly, the application of an operator to extract the edge strength (e.g. gradient) and in many cases direction (angle).

Thirdly, the application of a statistical criterion either locally or globally to select those pixels likely to lie in the region of an edge.

Fourthly, a thinning stage where an edge line is determined from the ensemble of pixels likely to lie in the edge region selected after 'thresholding'.

The actual edge operators are usually very simple. The Robert's operator for example is a simple 2x2 filter of form:

$$\begin{bmatrix} 0 & 1 \\ -1 & 0 \end{bmatrix} \qquad \begin{bmatrix} 1 & 0 \\ 0 & -1 \end{bmatrix}$$

The Sobel and Prewitt operators are 3x3 filters of form:

$$\begin{bmatrix} 1 & C & 1 \\ 0 & 0 & 0 \\ -1 & -C & -1 \end{bmatrix} \qquad \begin{bmatrix} 1 & 0 & -1 \\ C & 0 & -C \\ 1 & 0 & -1 \end{bmatrix}$$

The value of C is 1 for the Prewitt operator and 2 for the Sobel.

The Wechsler gradient operator has the basic form of:

$$\begin{bmatrix} 2 & 3 & 0 & -3 & -2 \\ 3 & 8 & 0 & -8 & -3 \\ 4 & 16 & 0 & -16 & -4 \\ 3 & 8 & 0 & -8 & -3 \\ 2 & 3 & 0 & -3 & -2 \end{bmatrix}$$

Note that these operators must be applied twice in two orthogonal directions (e.g. horizontally and vertically) and the results combined (as for a complex number) to give amplitude and direction. Thus if $F_h(i,j)$ is the result of the convolution in one direction and $F_v(i,j)$ the result after having rotated the filter by 90 degrees, then AMP(i,j) the amplitude image, and ANG(i,j) the direction image are generated by:

$$AMP(i,j) = [\ F_h(i,j)^2 + F_v(i,j)^2\ ]^{1/2}$$

$$ANG(i,j) = Tan^{-1} [\ F_v(i,j)\ /\ F_h(i,j)\ ]$$

These matrices AMP and ANG are often combined with a second differential operator (for example a Laplacian LAP(i,j)) such that a resultant data set RES(i,j) is created of form:

$$RES(i,j) = AMP(i,j) + k\ .\ LAP(i,j)$$

where k is an appropriate weight, usually dependent on the object. A 5x5 Laplacian filter has weights:

$$\begin{bmatrix} 0 & 1 & 1 & 1 & 0 \\ 1 & -2 & -1 & -2 & 1 \\ 1 & -1 & -C & -1 & 1 \\ 1 & -2 & -1 & -2 & 1 \\ 0 & 1 & 1 & 1 & 0 \end{bmatrix}$$

Note that the basic form of a gradient operator is that of a ramp (going from negative values on one side to positive values on the other through zero in the middle), while the Laplacian or 2nd differential operator is basically 'V' shaped. It may be convenient to think of the Laplacian operator as being some form of matched filter (see below).

3. Tests and results using phantoms

The filters described above were applied to both simulated and 'real' phantoms. The simulated phantoms comprised superimposed discs of various sizes and activities with various signal - to-noise ratios. The 'success' of the algorithms were tested (after thinning and the extraction of a suitable continuous contour) by counting the number of pixels included which should have been excluded, and the number of pixels falsely excluded. The sum of these two values gave an indication of the quality of the edge detecting algorithm for an object of constant size. Similar tests were performed for scans of active cylinders of known size and position. Thus the various edge operators were tested for their accuracy in finding the area of a region as a function of signal-to-noise ratio.

Very briefly the results were as follows:

1. The Laplacian operator was so sensitive at normal radioisotope signal - to-noise ratios that proper thinning was not obtained. It could not be tested adequately.

2. The Robert's operator was the least robust gradient operator in terms of poor performance at low signal-to-noise ratios.

3. The Sobel and Prewitt operators had similar performance and were less sensitive to poor signal-to-noise ratio.

3. The Wechsler was the least sensitive to signal-to-noise ratio, but tended to overestimate size.

In summary, the bigger the filter, the better the performance with respect to signal - to - noise ratio, but the greater the imprecision in finding the actual edge (as a result of the size of the filter).

Fig. 4. The results of
two different edge det-
ection operators (the
Sobel on the right and
the Prewitt on the left).
Almost no difference is
seen.

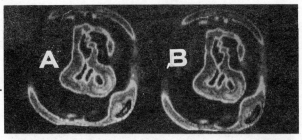

Fig. 5. For the profile
shown above, the lower
figure shows data
corresponding to the
chosen slice. The
three curves show the
raw data, a (signed)
gradient and the
second differential.
Note the absence of
a gradient peak in the
region of the spectrum
(arrowed) while there
is a very clear peak
in the second
differential.

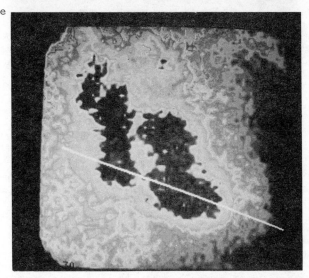

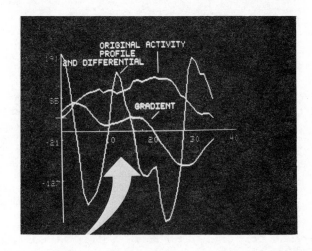

4. Results on clinical heart studies.

It was decided to test these various algorithms on a suitable set of clinical data. Fig. 2 shows an ensemble of 15 consecutive end-diastolic (ED) frames. Fig. 3 shows the result of applying the Wechsler operator to these images. It should be noted that the results obtained when using other gradient operators were nearly indistinguishable, as shown in Fig. 4. Certain general conclusions can be drawn. The 'outer' edge of the LV is in general well defined. There is, however, very poor determination of the inter-ventricular septum. It is not just that the algorithms perform poorly in this region, but more that (as seen in Fig. 4) there is very little gradient information associated with the septum. In general there is a well defined edge associated with high gradient values on the outer edges of both the right and left ventricles, and some rather poor information associated with the 'inner' edges of both right and left ventricles and very little associated with the septum as such.

In summary, it seems that the results obtained on phantom data cannot be extended to use with such clinical data. The situation is much more complex.

5. An alternative algorithm

It is of interest to look more closely at what is actually happening and what the data really convey . To this end sets of thick profiles at various angles through the LV were obtained, together with their gradient and 2nd differential. An example is shown in Fig. 5. Note that the one dimensional gradient is signed, whereas the gradient images, AMP(i,j), only show the absolute (positive) value of the 2-D gradient. The 1-D gradient shown here looks much smoother and cleaner. Similarly, the 2nd differential appears to be relatively noise free, and gives a large signal both for the 'outer' edges of RV and LV also for the septum. In this latter case, the concept of the 2nd differential operator as a kind of matched filter is very helpful in deciding the size and shape of the filter to be used, and the operator selected was chosen on these grounds. A mismatch of filter size and septum size will degrade the results.

In fact, for use of zoomed cardiac studies in a 64x64 matrix format, the gradient operator used was of form

$$[\quad -6 \quad -5 \quad -4 \quad -3 \quad -2 \quad -1 \quad 0 \quad 1 \quad 2 \quad 3 \quad 4 \quad 5 \quad 6 \quad]$$

and the 2nd differential operator had weights

$$[\quad 22 \quad 11 \quad 2 \quad -5 \quad -10 \quad -13 \quad -14 \quad -13 \quad -10 \quad -5 \quad 2 \quad 11 \quad 22 \quad]$$

The width of the profile used was 5 pixels, and thus the equivalent 2-D filters were 5x13 which are very large. It is for this reason that the 1-D filtered curves seem to be so noise free.

This suggested the following algorithm (which at the time was believed to be original):

1. Locate the 'centre' of the LV.

2. Obtain radial profiles at some suitable angular increment though the LV, e.g. convert to polar coordinates.

3. Obtain gradient and 2nd differentials of these profiles and detect maxima and minima.

4. Apply suitable constraints such that, for example, the max/min value of the gradient must lie within the max of the 2nd differential.

5. Apply radial smoothing (and possibly temporal constraints from cardiac images before and after the image being processed) and convert into a regular region of interest.

A number of other authors have published results using 2nd differential operators for cardiac edge detection, notably Goris (1980) and Almasi et al (1979). For comparison, the algorithm as described by Goris (1980) was tested on the same set of heart images. Unfortunately, the results were rather unsatisfactory in that rarely, with this set of data, were 'reasonable' LV outlines obtained (judged subjectively). It is likely that the explanation of these poor results lies in the small size of the Laplacian filter, being a one-dimensional filter of weights

[2   2   -2   -4   -2   2   2]

applied vertically, horizontally and diagonally. Such an algorithm can perhaps be made more stable by suitable preprocessing. However, it appears that, working in polar coordinates, a very convenient description of the LV is obtained, as will be described in the next section. Hawman (1979) described a technique using a combined gradient and Laplacian operator, this seems to have no intrinsic advantage over the methods described in the initial section, and did not appear to work on the type of data used for testing.

It cannot be stressed too much that many algorithms will perform satisfactorily when they are tested on small 'well-behaved' cardiac images, but 'fall to pieces' when tested on more complex abnormal studies. The method as developed by Verba (in Almasi et al 1979), as far as can be determined from the very brief description published, seems to correspond very closely to the method described here. A minor difference is that he used 48 radial profiles while, in this study, only 36 such profiles were obtained. However, tests indicated that the method is very insensitive to the angular sampling used.

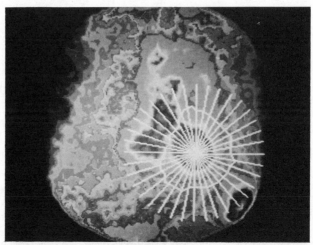

Fig. 6. A set of radial profiles with, super-imposed, a line joining the peaks in the second differential. The contour is the raw second differential region of interest.

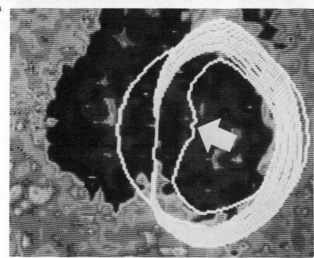

Fig. 7. A set of region of interest boundaries. The smallest ROI, shown arrowed, is the pure gradient ROI. The rest range from a pure second differential, to one which is pure gradient on the right, and pure second differential on the left. Also shown is the outer circle for locating the LV.

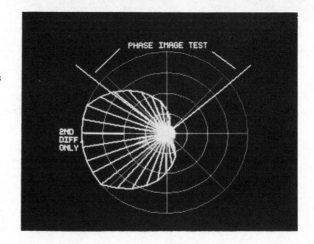

Fig. 8. The angular weights used for generating the set of ROIs shown in Fig. 7 above. The length of the radius distance as a function of angle is the weight given to the second differential. Also shown is the angle within which tests of the phase image are performed.

The centre of the LV was in fact determined manually by
placing a circle over the area identified as the LV. This gave an initial
estimate of the centre and size of the LV. The algorithm described is
relatively insensitive to imprecision in this first estimate. An automatic
algorithm, using information from the phase image and some crude
segmentation can provide such an estimate without operator intervention (e.g. in 'batch' mode).

6. Development of the algorithm

When radial contours are plotted, as shown in Fig. 6, the 2nd
differential contour appears to be very large outside the LV, whilst well
defining the ventricular septum. For this reason, the algorithm described
here has incorporated into it a set of radial weighting functions. At any
given angle, the radial distance to the 2nd differential and gradient
contour is determined. The final radial distance of the ROI contour is
obtained by interpolation between these two distances. Thus, the observer
selects a certain (maximum) weight for the gradient contour. A suitable
value seems to be 60%. Then, for the outer contour, a distance 60% away
from the 2nd differential contour towards the gradient contour is used.
The weight of the 2nd differential contour is increased towards the
ventricular septum, and becomes a pure 2nd differential contour in that
region. This is very convenient when the basic decription is in polar
coordinates. Note that the angle between the centre of gravity of the LV
and the RV seems to define the central angle of the septum in a
satisfactory manner. Fig. 7 shows a set of ROI contours ranging from a
pure gradient contour to a pure 2nd differential contour. Fig. 8 shows the
angular weighting function used.

Fig. 8 shows this radial weighting function balancing gradient and
2nd differential contour, together with a second (binary) weighting
function used to indicate that a test of the phase image (or to be
precise the cosine image) is to be made. Since a general problem is the
satisfactory definition of the valve plane, is is suggested that the phase
image contains useful relevant information. The algorithm tested was as
follows:

1. The (r,theta) coordinate of a point on the ROI
contour , if the value of theta is classed as being in the
region of the valve plane, is converted to an (x,y)
coordinate.

2. If the value of the phase image at that point shows a
'non-ventricular'   phase,   the   radial   distance   is
decremented.

3. The initial test is repeated while the radial distance
remains greater than some minimum distance.

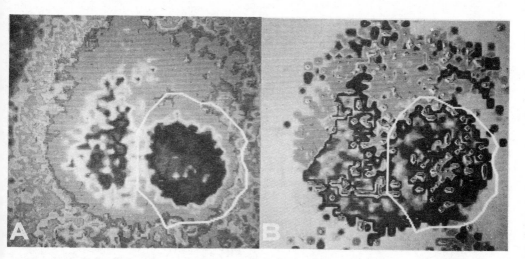

Fig. 9. On the left, the second differential ROI superimposed on the normal cardiac image and, on the right, superimposed on the phase image. Note that while this ROI appears to be too large in the normal image, it appears to be correct in the phase image.

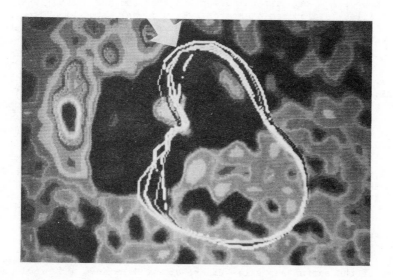

Fig. 10. Shows a set of ROIs from successive frames of a gated study superimposed on the phase image of a grossly abnormal patient. The dark area shows normal phase in the left and right ventricles. The approximate area of the valve plane is shown arrowed. The bottom region of the LV is an enormous aneurism.

Thus, a suitable constraint such that atrial regions are not included is easily added in polar coordinates. Note that the 'zero' phase region does <u>not</u> define the valve plane as such, it merely indicates when ventricular and atrial dynamic information are equal. Secondly, it is important not to include information from the phase image at other angles, since dyskinetic and akinetic regions should be included in the LV ROI and as such a test might exclude them on grounds of phase. In general, except in such cases, a reasonable match is found between the 2nd differential contour and the outer edge of the ventricle as observed in the phase image, (Fig. 9).

However many observers suggest that this contour is too large as a result of scatter and cardiac motion. It is for this reason that adding a certain bias from the gradient contour seems to be of value. The danger of using phase information indiscriminately is illustrated in Fig. 10, which shows superimposed onto the phase image of a patient with a large aneurism, the contours from a series of frames determined using the algorithm described above. Only phase information from the region of the valve plane has been incorporated. If the phase image had been used elsewhere in defining the LV region of interest, a grossly erroneous result would have been obtained.

7. Results

Most of the algorithms tested performed very poorly on difficult clinical material. For this reason, an algorithm based on extraction of radial profiles, and determination of gradient and 2nd differential on these profiles is proposed. Tests on 35 clinical studies have so far indicated very high stability with few problems occurring. The protocol used permits an observer to modify the LV ROI if desired. This has not been required.

Validation of the ROI contours produced by such algorithms is very difficult. While reliable determination of contours from frame to frame of a cardiac study is obtained, and even gives confidence that such contours could be used to study wall-motion (not an aim of the algorithm as such), there is no indication that the size of the final region of interest is optimal. Values of ejection fraction obtained using this algorithm are reasonable, but are they optimal? While they are precise, is there any bias? This can only be determined by comparison to other imaging modalities and clinical follow up. Such a clinical study has been initiated.

8. Background subtraction

All such algorithms require some form of background subtraction. However, if the septum and valve planes are well defined and provided an exact background correction is made, the determination of the outer contour of the LV is of no importance, provided it is big enough. ROI determination and background subtraction are linked. For example, the influence of the accuracy of the background subtraction is greater when a single ROI is used, than when the (more conventional) dual ED ES ROI technique is used (Fig. 11).

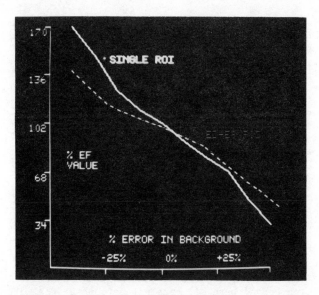

Fig. 11. The variation in EF as a function of the error made in the
background estimate for the single region of interest method (continuous
curve) and for the method of using ED and ES regions of interest (dotted
curve). The slope is greater for the single ROI technique showing that
the likely error is greater.

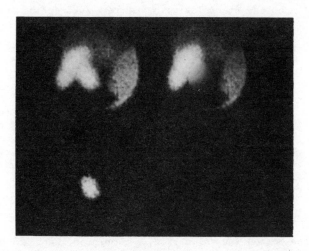

Fig. 12. The background subtration technique used for 'isolating' the
left ventricle. Above left is shown the raw data, above right is shown
the result of removing the LV, and below left is shown the isolated LV.
Note the variation in background in the area of the excised LV.

The technique   of background subtraction most commonly used   is
to place a horse-shoe shaped background region about the apex of the LV.
This can easily be generated automatically using the above (RPF) algorithm
However, an alternative approach using a more sophisticated background
subtraction is apparent.   This uses   the contour defined by the RPF
algorithm for the LV edge to produce estimates for background everywhere
within the LV region by interpolation.

This alternative technique determines BGD(i,j), the estimate of
background at a point (i,j) within the LV ROI using the form:

$$BGD(i,j) = \frac{\sum_{theta} WEIGHT(r,theta) \cdot EDGE(theta)}{\sum_{theta} WEIGHT(r,theta)}$$

where EDGE(theta) is a set of estimates of the background at the edge of
the ROI and WEIGHT(r,theta) is a suitable weighting function. The types of
weighting function tested were all simple functions of the distance from
the point (i,j) to the edge element, L. The types of function tested were:

1. $1/L$
2. $1/L^2$
3. $\exp(-L)$
4. $\exp(-L^2)$

Results of such an interpolative background subtraction are shown in
Fig. 12; above left is the raw data and above right is the result of
subtracting the LV.   Using this technique, an isolated LV can be
obtained   from which the EF can be estimated merely by summing the total
LV counts.

Thus, the following types of background subtraction were tested on
clinical and phantom data:-
1. A standard horseshoe surrounding the LV (determined
automatically).
2. An interpolative background estimate such that every point
within the LV ROI has a value determined by a combination of all
edge values, after correction for Compton scatter, using a $1/L^2$
function.

9. The simulated model of the heart

As a further method for validation, a simulated cardiac model was
designed and used. This comprised four chambers defined by ellipsoids of
rotation for which, as a function of time, the centre, angles of rotation
and tilt, and sizes of the various axes could be controlled. The formation
of the model then comprised the following steps:

1. Generation of the pure ellipsoids with variable size position
etc as shown in Fig. 13.
2. Blurring by the collimator response function (assumed to be
Gaussian), addition of random noise and scatter, as shown in
Fig. 14.

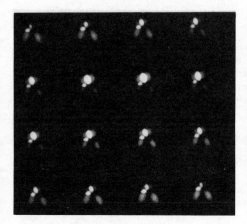

Fig. 13. The original
ellipsoids of rotation for
the set of 16 frames of the
gated study.

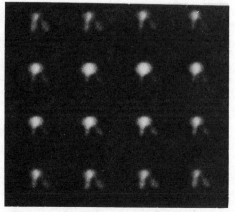

Fig. 14. The set of data after
blurring with the collimator
response function.

Fig. 15. The final result of adding
background to represent other background structures and Poisson noise.

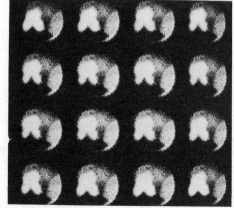

Fig. 16. Pairs of ED and ES
images from a set of simulations
with various known ejection
fractions ranging from 11.5%, top
left, to 71.5, bottom right.

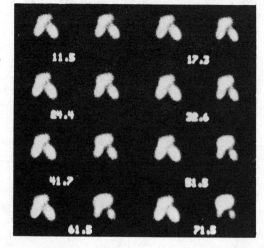

3. Addition of 'coloured' background as shown in Fig. 15.
From this a set of studies could be created as shown in Fig. 16. Here, pairs of ED and ES images are shown for a set of data with <u>known</u> EF, varying from 5% to 75%. Several such sets of data were generated which formed the model test set for the evaluation.

10. Results using the model and clinical data.

Regressions were performed for the four techniques tested and the correlation coefficient r determined:

1. Radial Filtered Profiles (RPF) with a horseshoe background: with r=0.8
2. RPF with an interpolated $1/L^2$ background: with r=0.75
3. Laplacian ROI with manual value plane definition: with r=0.78
4. Laplacian ROI with automatic value plane definition: with r=0.83

While there is little difference in significance, the RPF algorithm gave a regression line which is much closer to the line of identity; the Laplacian technique consistently underestimated EF.

When tested against the model, the RPF technique gave a correlation coefficient of 0.98.

These results should be compared with those reported by Nalcioglu who showed, when comparing the angiographic length-breadth technique with that of digital radiography (i.e. integration of contrast within an LV ROI), that on the same image a correlation coefficient of 0.96 could be obtained while on the same study a correlation coefficient of 0.94 was obtained. Isotopic techniques must therefore expect an r of less than this last value. There are (at least) two hypotheses to explain these results: that radio-isotopic angiography is inaccurate and the model results are so good because the model is unrealistic, or the alternative, that the angiographic 'gold standard' is inappropriate. It is suggested that the latter hypothesis is more realistic. In summary, the correlation with the model is much better than for true angiographically validated clinical data, probably because of errors in estimating 'true' EF.

11. Conclusion

In conclusion, while this study does not claim to present any new or revolutionary algorithms for use with cardiac images, it is intended to illustrate the dangers of blindly using techniques developed in the general image processing field, and applying them without thought to the rather curious data found in nuclear medicine. Probably the success of the radial profile algorithm can be attributed to the fact that it is highly constrained. Implicitly, a well-specified model of the LV region has been assumed. In many nuclear medicine image processing applications, the greater the amount of incorporated a-priori information, the greater the likelihood of satisfactory results. Such use of a priori information is one method to enable 'sophisticated' image processing techniques to be used with the very poor quality data which seems to exist in radioisotope studies.

Acknowledgments

The clinical material tested was obtained at the Hopital Beaujon, Clichy, France, and the author would like to acknowledge in particular the support of Dr. F. Cavailloles and other clinical colleagues, as well as of C.W. Kwok and Hugh Duncan of UCL Dept. of Computer Science, who assisted with the program development.

References

Almasi J.J., Bornstein I., Eisner R.L., Goliash T.J., Nowak D.J., Verba J.W., Enhanced clinical utility of nuclear cardiology through advanced computer processing methods, Proc. Symp. 'Computers in Cardiology', Geneva 1979, in press, (available as reprint from GE Milwaukee Wis 53201).

Bossuyt A., Deconinck F., Lepoudre R., Jonckheer M., The temporal Fourier transform as applied to functional isotopic imaging, in 'Information Processing in Medical Imaging', Les Colloques de l'INSERM 88 Paris (1980), 88.

Cahill P.T., Ornstein E., Ho S.L., Edge detection algorithms in nculear medicine, IEEE Trans. NS NS-23 , (1976), 555.

Geffers H., Adam W.E., Bitter F., Sigel H., Kampmann H., Data processing and functional imaging in radionuclide ventriculography, in 'Information Processing in Medical Imaging', ORNL-BTCIC-2 (1977), 322.

Goris M.L., Briandet Ph.A., Huffer E., Edge tracing algorithms in nuclear medicine, Proc. WAMI Versailles (1980), in press.

Hawman E.G., Digital boundary detection techniques for the analysis of gated cardiac scintigrams, SPIE Vol 206 , 'Recent and future developments in medical imaging II', (1979), 224.

Levialdi S., Finding the edge, in 'Digital Image Processing and Analysis', NATO ASI, (INRIA, Rocquencourt France, 1980), 167.

Pratt W.K., 'Digital Image Processing', (Wiley, New York, 1978), Chapter 17.

Rosenfeld A., Thurston M., Edge and curve detection for visual scene analysis, IEEE Trans. Computers C-20 ,5, (1971), 562.

Zadeh L.A., Biological applications of the theory of fuzzy sets, in 'Biocybernetics of the nervous system', (Little Brown and Co., Boston Mass., 1970).

Radiological Techniques in Cardiology: An Overview

B M Moores

Regional Department of Medical Physics, Christie Hospital, Withington, Manchester, M20 9BX.

Abstract

Cardiac radiology is used to study both heart function and form and important considerations in any overview of this subject are:-

a)   The anatomical sites and structures involved.

b)   The radiological techniques employed.

c)   The technological developments which form the foundation of modern cardiac radiology.

The evolution of this branch of radiology has been intimately related to the technological developments occurring in all aspects of X-ray equipment.   Consequently, developments in X-ray tube, generator, image intensifier/TV systems, image recording, manipulation and display systems have all contributed to the existing capabilities of cardiac radiology.

1.   Introduction.

Vascular diseases in general and those involving the heart in particular are one of the major problems facing the health care industry in Western societies.   For instance, approximately 50 per cent of all annual deaths in the United Kingdom may be directly attributed to vascular diseases with 65 per cent of these due to diseases of the heart.   Cardiological investigations, therefore, play an important role in modern medical practice and together with surgical intervention often lead to a significant improvement in quality of life.

Radiological techniques are an important component in the overall cardiological spectrum, particularly when it is desirable to correlate visual aspects of function and form with other physiological data. The historical development of radiology in cardiology originates almost from the time of Roentgen's initial discovery and has been presented previously (Steiner 1973).   However, such is the pace of technical development, new radiological techniques have appeared within the past decade.   Consequently, the modern catheterization laboratory is radiologically different from earlier laboratories although the essential features of the equipment are still the same.

An overview of radiological techniques in cardiology should first of all
be concerned with the anatomy involved since these can greatly
influence the radiological requirements necessary to undertake a
useful investigation.   Secondly, because a wide spectrum of radiological
techniques can be employed, depending upon the nature of the investigation, these also need outlining.   Finally, because of constant
improvements, modifications or development of new techniques, the
technical developments which have been instrumental in this progress
are worth consideration.

2. Anatomical Structures

The heart maintains the blood circulation throughout the body supplying
two main components, the pulmonary and systemic circulation.   The
pulmonary circulation is fed by the right ventricle via the pulmonary
arteries, the oxygenated blood returning to the left atrium.   The
pulmonary circuit is of low pressure with the lungs offering little
resistance to flow.   Oxygenated blood is pumped by the left ventricle
into the systemic circulation returning back to the right atrium.
Because many circulatory diseases involve both the peripheral circulation as well as the heart itself it is not always possible to separate
cardiological investigations from peripheral vascular studies.

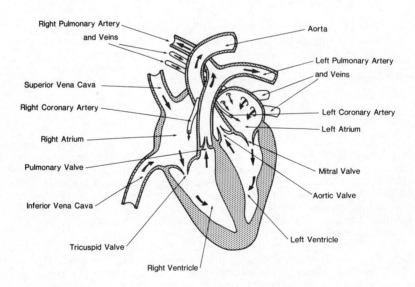

Figure 1   Schematic outline of the heart.

Although there are obvious links between pulmonary or peripheral circulation and cardiac function the cardiological applications of
radiology may be confined to the heart itself and the immediately
adjacent vessels.   The heart, shown schematically in Fig. 1, comprises

four chambers separated by the tricuspid, pulmonary, aortic and mitral
valves.   During both contraction (systole) and relaxation (diastole)
phases of the heart   anatomical motion of up to 400 mm/sec are not
uncommon (Jensen and Kuntke, 1967).   Consequently, any detailed study
of structures within the heart will require extremely short exposure
times to minimise motion blurring.   Also, because of the complexity
of structures involved and the close proximity of the heart to the spine
it is desirable to be able to view the heart from more than one
direction.

Although the large vessels entering and leaving the heart are relatively
large, the coronary arteries which supply the heart itself with blood
have relatively small diameters, particularly some way from the main
branch.   Radiological investigation of coronary artery disease, therefore, does require satisfactory contrast and spatial resolution.
Indeed, the ability to detect moving edges also has similar requirements.
Because of the stringent imaging requirements of certain investigations,
the expansion of radiology into these areas has followed closely behind
technical developments.

Radiology is now employed as a major diagnostic tool in investigations
of both degenerative or acquired and congenital defects associated with
most of the heart's major structures.   It is employed in investigations
involving stenosis, valvular insufficiency, ischemia and septal defects.
Congenital heart disease can be investigated radiographically from the
earliest time and involves a wide range of defects.   Radiology is
employed in investigations of both function and form providing both
pathological and physiological information.   The evolution of physiological measurements is based upon dynamic studies.   The ability to
measure, quantitatively, changes in flow provides useful additional
information.   However, the radiologist's ability to correlate radiological changes with other physiological data also provides a qualitative physiological component .

Acquired heart disease may occur in late childhood and throughout adult
life, whilst congenital diseases occur at birth.   Cardiac radiology
applies, therefore, to the whole age spectrum which itself produces a
wide range of radiographic requirements.   Besides being a purely
diagnostic modality it is also employed as an investigative technique
following surgical intervention in valve replacement or graft patency
studies.

The radiographic techniques employed depend upon the age of the patient
or the nature of the disease.   It is true to say, however, that
virtually the whole spectrum of techniques are applied ranging from
plain film to CT scanning.   The range of techniques employed are as
follows:-

> Plain film
> Plain film   - angiography
> Fluoroscopy   - catheter location
> Fluoroscopy   - angiography
>   arteriography
> Computer image analysis - quantitative studies
> Computer assisted tomography
> Digital fluoroscopy.

3. Radiographic Techniques

3.1. Plain Film

Conventional radiographs of the chest are extremely useful in evaluating the lungs, the size of the heart, cardiac chambers and main
vascular connections to the heart.   Because the heart and lungs are
closely related geographically and hemodynamically then lung vasculature can provide useful information regarding cardiac function. For
instance, increased pulmonary blood flow resulting from shunts within
the heart.   These can lead to relatively high pulmonic-systemic blood
flow ratios.   This simple radiographic technique is also extremely
useful when there is a need to wait and see before more detailed
investigations may be undertaken.

3.2. Serial Plain Film

Multiple rapid sequence plain film studies in conjunction with the
injection of contrast material still has a significant role to play in
routine cardiological investigations.   Between 5 and 10 images can be
accommodated during a single cardiac cycle or alternatively physiological gating can provide images at predetermined points in the cycle.
One advantage of this technique is the high resolution images which
can be produced since normally film/screen combinations have higher
resolution than image intensifier systems, the alternative method of
producing rapid sequence images.

3.3. Fluoroscopy - Catheter Localization

An integral part of modern cardiac investigations involves selective
positioning of a catheter in order to undertake physiological monitoring
or inject contrast material.   For instance, selective dextro and levo
cardiography, pulmonal and coronary arteriography provide contrast
investigations of particular parts of the cardiac anatomy without the
complications of other structural detail.   The use of specially shaped
catheters for accurate tip localization in the coronary arteries, and
the Sones and Judkins techniques has helped to make coronary arteriography a routine procedure.   Fluoroscopic imaging plays a major role
in the catheterization procedure.

3.4. Fluoroscopy - Angiography/Arteriography

The most widely used radiological technique in cardiological investigations is cine angiography employing image intensifier detection.
The basic components of the system are shown in Fig. 2.   The output
from the intensifier is fed either to a TV camera or a cine camera by
means of a beam splitting device.   Whilst preparing for contrast
injection fluoroscopy only the TV camera is employed.

On injection of the contrast agent the X-ray output is increased and
synchronized with a cine camera, usually operated in the region of
30-50 frames per second.   High quality film recording of the movement
of contrast material in the heart and major vessels provides the
radiologist with structural and dynamic detail.

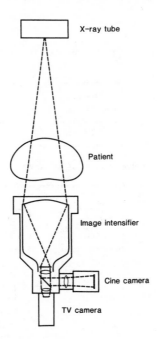

Figure 2   Image intensifier/TV system for cine-angiography

With the advent of video tape recorders this form of image storage is
also used to store the signal from the TV camera.   This method provides
the radiologist with instant playback and freeze frame capability but
with poorer image quality than cine film.   Cine-angiography is an
extremely useful investigative technique in diseases of the coronary
artery and myocardium, some valvular disorders, septal defects and
diseases of the major vessels.   Similarly, following surgical intervention in coronary artery disease, graft patency can be investigated by
this technique.

3.5.   Quantitative Studies

Visual observation of plain films, cine films or video tape images provides a subjective appraisal of heart function.   In order to provide
objective interpretation more detailed analysis is required.   The basic
components of quantitative evaluation are shown in Fig. 3.   The
X-ray image is analyzed densitometrically and, having selected particular
regions of interest, two forms of measurement can be undertaken.   First,
by locating equal density regions, the edges of the heart or individual
chambers can be determined.   Then, by measuring changes in position with
time, either area or computed volume changes can be calculated.   Alternatively, evaluation of the average brightness in well defined regions
enables determination of the computed flow and flow-rates.

Quantitative data provide a more detailed analysis of radiological
information and by correlating this information with other physiological

data provide   a broad based assessment of cardiac function.

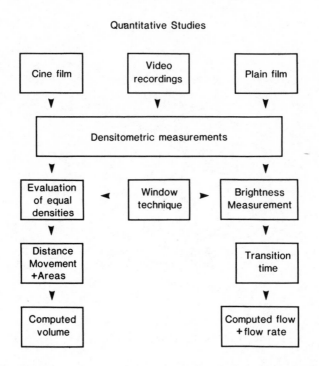

Figure 3   Main components of quantitative image analysis

3.6. CT Scanning

Over the past ten years the evolution of CT technology has been towards
faster scan times.   This has led to the facility to perform rapid
image reconstructions in a plane through which contrast agent is
flowing.   By measuring changes in the CT number values, flow through
major vessels can be computed.   In order to perform the rapid image
sequence following contrast injection a fast scan is undertaken in one
direction.   After a brief inter-scan period the procedure is repeated
in the reverse direction.   Interlaced images are then reconstructed
using segments of the single scan data.   This results in flow curves
which it is hoped will provide useful additional hemodynamic information.
At the present time this technique is largely confined to the major
vessels.   However, with the development of multiple X-ray tube or scanned
electron beam X-ray sources, the potential for extremely rapid image
reconstructions could lead to dynamic three-dimensional investigations.

3.7. Digital Fluoroscopy

Digital fluoroscopy combines fluoroscopic angiography with computerized
quantitative image analysis to provide on-line data processing which
offers some interesting angiographic possibilities.   These systems

digitize the video signal from the TV camera and store the data in some
form of digital memory sub-system.   On-line manipulation of the data
provides the facility to integrate frames hence reducing noise, subtract
images hence reducing structural noise, or produce time interval
difference studies.

Image subtraction reduces the dynamic range of the detected transmitted
variations, so that extremely low contrasts can be optimally displayed
providing maximum visual appreciation.   In order to ensure low contrast
perceptibility, quantum noise must be kept as low as possible which means
relatively high X-ray exposures, in fluoroscopic terms, must be employed.
To ensure that threshold contrast is quantum limited requires that the
noise generated in the imaging system is kept to a minimum, in particular
electronic noise in the TV camera/video amplifier chain.   The ability
to detect low contrasts using subtraction techniques has resulted in the
use of angiographic studies using intra-venous contrast injection.   Even
so, relatively large bolus injections are required and investigations
are limited to the major vessels including those of the heart.   Although
an extremely recent development, digital fluoroscopy has already undergone significant technical development and offers possibilities for new
types of investigation.   Nonetheless, digital fluoroscopy may be
employed routinely in cardiological investigations even with arterial
injections since the instantaneous visualization of subtracted images
could help to simplify diagnosis.

4. Historical Development

Radiological investigations of the heart date almost from the time of
Roentgen's initial discovery in 1895.   However, modern cardiac radiology may be traced to the late 1940's by which time the essential
features of modern investigations had emerged, namely catheterization,
contrast injection and serial imaging.   Since this time the scope of
radiological involvement in cardiology has continued to grow based upon
continued technical development in every aspect of X-ray equipment;
namely the tube, generator, image intensifier, TV system, data handling
and display.   Much of this development has been gradual, corresponding
to improvements in individual components of a particular piece of equipment.   A brief summary of this development helps to put into perspective
the existing capability of modern cardiological X-ray equipment.

4.1. X-ray Tube

The short-term loadability L of an X-ray tube is given by the expression:

$$L = K \frac{1}{\sin \alpha} \sqrt{bDn}$$

where l and b are the projected focal spot length and width, α the
target angle, D the mean diameter of the focal track, n the rotation
frequency and K a constant which depends upon the thermal properties of
the anode materials.   The long-term loadability of the tube is governed
by the anode size, specific heat and its ability to radiate heat.
Virtually every aspect of tube design which affects both short and long
term loadability has undergone constant development and refinement over
the past 20-30 years, particularly in the following key areas:-

a)   Anode construction - increased size, stress resistant shape, construction materials, surface colour, focal spot focusing

b) Anode rotation - increased speed, improved bearings.

c) Tube insert - materials other than glass in the walls.

d) Tube housing - forced cooling, air or water.

All these developments have led to tubes with the following characteristics:-

Focal Spots	0.6/1.3 mm
Rated power	50/150 kW
Anode heat)	
Storage capacity)	400 kW
Anode speed	8000 rpm
Disc diameter	120 mm
Disc weight	1 kg

Crack resistant design
Blackened anode

4.2. Generator

Generators have also undergone gradual improvements in all facets of operation.   Increased power through the use of 6 and 12 pulse three phase waveform and higher mA capabilities have led to shorter exposure times.   Improved stabilization and compensation facilities and automatic brightness and gain control circuits mean image quality is consistent.   The facility to employ pulsed operation with short exposure times reduces motion blurring and also ensures that dose efficiency is optimal.   External switching control provides physiological and/or contrast injection exposure control.   Finally, the advent of microprocessor control ensures that technique variability is comprehensive and easily controlled with minimum fault potential.

4.3. Image Intensifier

Image intensifier design has undergone rapid developments, particularly over the past 20 years.   The introduction of caesium iodide input phosphors has led to both higher and more uniform spatial resolution, improved X-ray detection and higher conversion efficiency.   Improvement in electron optics has also improved resolution , particularly its uniformity, and has led to larger field sizes.   The external housing has seen the introduction of new materials in the external front face to maintain strength but reduce X-ray absorption, also the use of non-magnetic materials to minimise its effect on the electron optics.   The output phosphor has shown improved light output as well as colour matching to film rather than eye response.   Finally, the optical coupling has been improved to ensure improved quantum transfer and resolution.

The evolution of digital fluoroscopic techniques, where minimum contrast detectability will always be a prime requirement, ensures that imaging capability is always operating at the upper limit of equipment performance.   Consequently, each small improvement in image intensifier technology leads to an overall improvement in system performance which helps to provide additional useful information.

4.4. Recording and Display

Although film is still the primary recording medium in angiographic
investigations, this too has undergone improvements.   It has been
better matched in terms of speed, contrast and resolution to the
fluorographic requirements.   Automatic brightness control ensures
optimum and consistent exposure whilst the intensifier light output
spectral matching has led to improvements in speed.   TV camera design
has been primarily aimed at meeting low exposure rate fluoroscopic
requirements.   However, with the evolution of digital fluoroscopy low
camera noise becomes important.   Consequently, a review of the most
desirable camera design, vidicon, plumbicon, etc., seems appropriate.
Also, scan speed, beam current and beam area are important.   The
advent of large format intensifiers will also place stringent requirements on camera resolution, particularly if accompanied by requirements
for low contrast detectability.

The advent of video tape and digital storage media are more recent but
nontheless have led to the facility of electronically enhancing the
displayed data.   For instance, the dynamic range compression which
follows subtraction enables the displayed signals to be amplified for
maximum visual contrast.   The architecture of digital fluoroscopic
systems has already undergone development since its recent emergence and
no doubt this will continue.

4.5. Equipment Configuration

Lateral and AP images have been employed routinely for a number of years
to ensure over or underlying structures do not obscure relevant detail.
The evolution of coronary arteriography led to more variable projection
capability.   Consequently C and U-arm assemblies now provide a wide
range of oblique caudal and cranial projections as well as the more
usual lateral and AP configuration.   This reduces the need to physically move the patient or table top cradle in order to achieve oblique
projections which can be an advantage when dealing with patients suffering from heart disease.

4.6. CT and Digital Systems

Developments within the CT framework have led to its application in
angiography.   Improvements in detector technology, configuration and
construction have improved resolution and reduced scan time.   Gantry
improvements have led to faster scans which are fundamental to dynamic
studies.   Data collection and manipulation has needed to develop to
provide the rapid reconstructions and ability to measure flow through
vessels.   Prospective developments in CT technology may, in fact, lead
to its overlap or development into digital radiography.

The recent emergence of digital fluoroscopic techniques has been built
upon developments in many facets of X-ray equipment.   However, it is
now spawning developments within its own framework.   Energy subtraction
for optimum visualization of particular anatomical detail as well as
spatial filtering techniques to accomodate bolus injection are
possibilities provided by the digital data handling.   The potential
to broaden fluoroscopy into general radiographic practice is also being
pursued and would provide all radiographic modalities outlined
previously within a single system.

References

Steiner R E   1973   Brit. J. Radiol. $\underline{46}$ 741
Jensen F and Kuntke A   1967   Medicamundi $\underline{12}$ 123

Theory and Practice of Applying Image Analysis to Angiography

J N H Brunt, C J Taylor, R N Dixon

Department of Medical Biophysics, University of Manchester, M13 9PT, U K

P J Gregory

Joyce-Loebl (Vickers PLC), Team Valley, Gateshead, NE11 0QW, U K

Abstract. Image acquisition facilities may be added to almost
any computer to permit digital image analysis. In practice, for
cases where the image is complex, and time and expense must be
limited, conventional computers have serious drawbacks. For
angiographic images, therefore, it is advantageous to employ a
computer system with an appropriately specialised architecture.
Important goals in the design of image analysis hardware are that
the system should be able to implement essential algorithms at
high speed and that it should facilitate application of this
enhanced performance to new problems as they are recognised. To
attain these joint goals, hardware and software must be
considered together. We describe how the Magiscan 2 image
analyser incorporates these concepts, and illustrate its
application to enhancement of sequences of images from left
ventriculograms, automated ventricular outline delineation, and
acquisition of information from sets of ventricular outlines.

1. Introduction

This paper is concerned with the application of digital systems in
analysing angiographic images. The amount of data contained in these
images favours the use of a computer system whose architecture has been
designed specifically for image manipulation. A general purpose
processor normally proves rather slow and it is often difficult to
arrange software in a way that allows new problems to be solved
efficiently. We shall describe an approach in which serial processing
is used but where the design of the architecture allows significant
improvements over the performance obtainable with a general purpose
serial computer.

Among design requirements, the importance of high processor performance
is equalled by that of the ability to express the solution of a problem
in a clear and concise manner. These requirements demand that the
hardware and software of a system evolve concurrently. We shall
describe the products of this evolution in the context of the Magiscan
2 image analysis system, which we have been involved in designing, and
shall discuss some specific examples of application.

2. Operations on images

As a starting point we should look at some of the types of operation
that it is important to be able to perform on images. Operations can be
divided into those that are essentially parallel and those that are
essentially serial. The division is of course arbitrary since with some
contortion it is possible to describe any operation in either way:
there is, however, a natural division.

Contrast manipulation and image arithmetic are examples of essentially
parallel operations. In contrast manipulation the same rule is applied
to each picture element (pixel), assigning new grey level values which
improve visual contrast by stretching or compressing appropriate
portions of the grey scale. Image arithmetic includes addition (where
grey levels from corresponding pixels in two or more images are added to
produce an averaged image), and subtraction (where subtraction of
corresponding pixels from two images can remove structures common to
both images). Figure 1 a) shows one frame from a left ventricular
cine-angiogram. If we perform image addition to average several frames
spanning the cardiac cycle prior to contrast injection, then subtract
the mask image so obtained from the image in Figure 1 a), we obtain an
image in which the conspicuity of the left ventricle is enhanced with
respect to that of other structures such as the diaphragm or ribs
(Figure 1 b)). If we subtract closely adjacent frames then the Time
Interval Difference image so obtained (Figure 1 c)) shows those regions
where contrast is entering or leaving pixels.

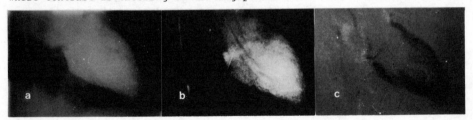

Fig. 1 Image manipulation of frames from a ventriculogram.
       (a) Original image. (b) Original with unopacified frame subtracted.
       (c) Original with preceding frame subtracted.

Searching and measurement are examples of essentially serial operations.
Searching could for example consist of finding the exact position of
some image feature starting from knowledge of its approximate position.
Measurement could be finding the length of a line or the area of a
shadow. The important property that these types of operation have in
common is that ordering is important and that is what makes them
essentially serial. We shall illustrate examples of serial operations
in a later section of the paper.

3. Software for Image Analysis

We suggested in the introduction that an important requirement of an image
analysis system is the ability to tackle new problems efficiently. In
practice this means that the system must be programmable in a high level
language. Furthermore, the high level language that is used should
support the different types of data structure that will be generated
during an analysis.

One of the types of data structure will be the IMAGE (this can be considered as simply a two dimensional array), and parallel operations will simply generate further IMAGEs. As an analysis progresses, however, we become interested in different data structures consisting of groups or sets of points. These can be described by the generic name POINTSET. We may be interested in single POINTs, in ARCs or closed BOUNDARY(s) that describe features of interest, or in solid areas: sometimes irregular REGIONs and sometimes rectangular WINDOWs. These variant forms of the data structure POINTSET are illustrated in Figure 2.

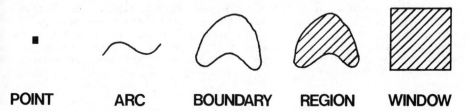

POINT   ARC   BOUNDARY   REGION   WINDOW

Fig. 2 Variant forms of the data structure POINTSET.

It is important that although the data describing these entities may be stored in computer memory in different forms they will tend to be used in similar ways. In particular they will often be used to apply an operation to an IMAGE. We have implemented a scheme based on the Pascal language (Jensen and Wirth 1975) with standard data structures and procedures to manipulate them.

4. Hardware for Image Analysis

The considerations in the previous sections have led us to define three design constraints on an image analysis system. Firstly, the system must manipulate the data structure IMAGE. Secondly, it must perform efficiently an important class of operations that involve treating each pixel identically, resulting in a new or transformed IMAGE: such manipulations (IMAGE to IMAGE transformations) are often called image processing. Thirdly, analysis involves transformations of IMAGEs into other data structures, and at this stage the ordering of the pixels is important.

Hence we have developed hardware to perform both image processing and image analysis efficiently. We have chosen a basically serial architecture because it is usually extremely difficult to use parallel architecture efficiently to perform serial tasks.

We can now list the elements required in the hardware. Firstly, memory for programs and data. To perform the types of IMAGE to IMAGE transformation we have mentioned we need to store multiple IMAGEs at approximately 256 x 256 pixels resolution, with at least 64 grey levels. Next, processing: we need to be able to perform arithmetic and logical operations on many different types of data. Next, addressing: one of the major operations involved in manipulating structured data is that of computing memory addresses to access the data elements. In image processing, address computation for numerous pixels can be as important as the data processing. Finally, input/output: provision must be made for image loading and display, and for other forms of user interaction.

The system that evolved from these considerations is illustrated in its commercially-available form in Figure 3, and its block diagram is shown in Figure 4. The only element of the system not contained in the desktop console is the TV camera used for image input. Current technology has allowed us to place all the elements such as processors in a small volume behind the TV display. The block diagram shows that at the centre of the system is the Image Memory. This is kept separate from a general purpose Program and Data Memory. An Arithmetic and Logic Processor (ALP), which can manipulate data in either memory, is included. There is a special processor to compute image memory addresses (MAP). The ALP and MAP are controlled in sychronism by the Microprogrammed Controller. Image input and display are in real—time direct into and out of the Image Memory. Programmable lookup tables allow, for example, logarithmic transformation of incoming image intensity values. A TV camera is the normal input device, but other devices or methods of image acquisition can be used.

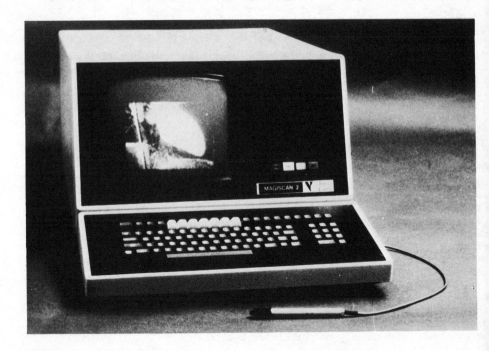

Fig. 3 Magiscan 2 image analysis system, in its production form.

Figure 5 shows how the system can exhibit different personalities. The grouping of Microprogram Controller, ALP, Program + Data Memory and I/O Controller is basically a modern minicomputer capable of executing high level language programs. The video I/O and Image Memory together form a raster graphics display system. The group of Microprogram Controller, ALP, MAP and Image Memory is an image processor capable of high speed image to image transformations.

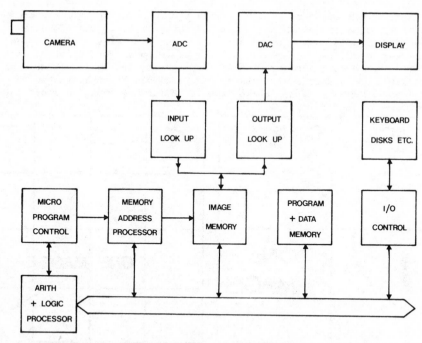

Fig. 4 Block diagram of the Magiscan 2 image analysis system.

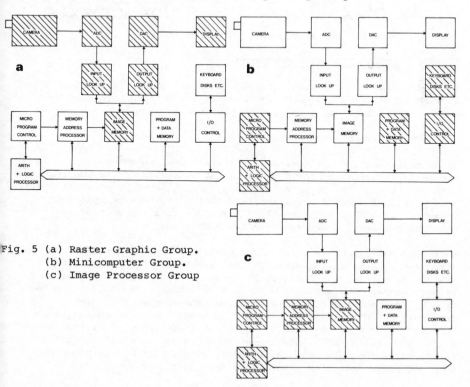

Fig. 5 (a) Raster Graphic Group.
(b) Minicomputer Group.
(c) Image Processor Group

The Image Memory or Store is 1024 pixels square. Each pixel is stored
as 8 bits, so an image can have up to 256 grey-levels. The store is
expandable to 1024 square by 16 bits. Images of fewer than 8 bits can
be stacked on top of one another. Alternative modes for using the store
are as 4 images of 512 square, or as 16 images of 256 square (Figure 6).
This last mode is particularly useful for analysis of angiographic
sequences. With the expansion to 16 bits, 32 images could be stored at
8 (or fewer) bits of course.

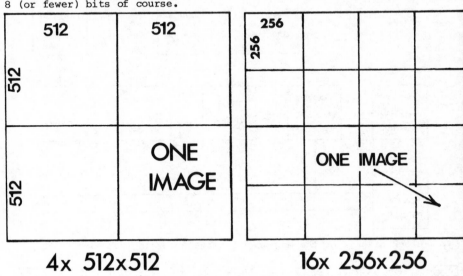

Fig. 6 Alternative modes for using the image store

5. Application to Cardioangiography

In this section we describe the image analysis tasks that need to be
tackled in cardioangiography, and explain how the approach that we have
adopted facilitates solution of the problems involved.

5.1 Ventricular Outline Delineation

In automated outline delineation, the first goal is accuracy - to avoid
the need for manual correction, as far as possible. It is important to
remember that manual verification (and correction where necessary) will
occupy several seconds per frame, and that therefore the speed of
detection will only significantly affect the total time involved if more
than several seconds are required for each frame.

There are two separable cases of automatic boundary detection. In the
first case, catheter angiography, the algorithms used depend upon
whether or not image processing is used. Without image processing, such
as subtraction, our experience is that reliability can only be achieved
by building into the program projection-dependent morphological
information. With image processing, however, the enhanced images
obtained (Figure 1) may permit projection-independent algorithms to be
used. The second case, intravenous angiography (which of necessity
incorporates image processing) involves superimposed structures that
make automatic detection a much more difficult problem.

Before the advent of whole-image processing, several groups (e.g.Barrett
et al 1980, Slager et al 1978) described systems for automatic outline
detection: these systems were applied to catheter angiography without
subtraction. We developed a software package using algorithmic elements
typical of these systems (Brunt et al 1979). In the first frame of the
angiographic sequence, partial manual initialization is used: the
operator indicates five single POINTs on the outline. As shown in Figure
7, these POINTs are the two margins of the aortic valve, the apex and a
position on the inferior and on the anterior wall of the ventricle. From
these five POINTs the computer draws the initial model BOUNDARY as a
succession of ARCs. This merely determines the REGION for the outline
search, which then follows automatically.

In subsequent frames, the preceding BOUNDARY is used as a model to speed
the detection process by limiting the search range. The outline detection
process employs information of two kinds: first, predictive information
derived from orientations, curvatures and speeds of motion of the BOUNDARY
in earlier frames, and second, edge information such as density
gradients in the grey levels of the image. An example of an automatically
delineated BOUNDARY is shown in Figure 8.

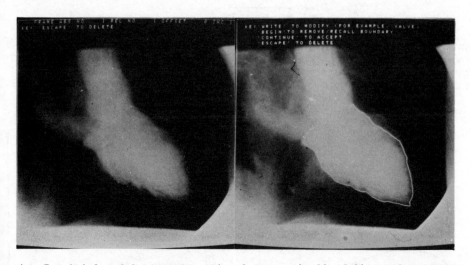

Fig. 7 Initial model BOUNDARY. Fig. 8 Automatically delineated BOUNDARY

5.2 Obtaining Information from Ventricular Outlines

We shall now look at what kinds of information can be obtained, from a
sequence of ventricular outlines, using image analysis. First, assuming
that some distance calibration technique is available, measurements or
estimates of time varying quantities such as volume can be made. From
these quantities, it is then possible to calculate indices of the overall
function of the ventricle: obvious examples are ejection fraction and
peak systolic ejection rate. The second type of information obtainable
is that for segmental outline motion analysis. The different types of
information will be discussed in the following paragraphs.

Ventricular volume can be estimated either using geometrical models or by densitometric techniques. The latter techniques are only feasible if image processing has been used. The processing consists of logarithmic transformation of intensity values to relative density values, followed by subtraction of a pre-injection image (mask image). The next requirement is good mixing of blood and contrast medium. Even if this can be achieved, incorrect values will still be obtained unless a correction is applied for radiation scattering and intensifier glare.

In view of the difficulties mentioned in the last paragraph, we may expect most volume estimates to continue to be done using any of a number of geometrical models. An ellipsoid of revolution (Figure 9) is most commonly used as a first approximation to the ventricular shape. For single-plane films the depth of the ventricle is then assumed to be equal to the width (that is, minor axis) of an ellipse of area equal to the measured area in the observed projection. Finally, the longest axis of the ventricle is used as the major axis of the ellipsoid. The volume can then be expressed by the simple formula:

$$\text{Volume} = \frac{8 \times (\text{Area})^2}{3 \times \pi \times \text{Length}}$$

This first approximation gives a systematic overestimation of volume, so empirical regression equations are then used to get a better approximation. Figure 10 shows graphs of volume and its first derivative over a period slightly longer than one cardiac cycle. In drawing graphs, the availability of variants, such as ARCs and WINDOWs, of the data structure POINTSET is particularly welcome.

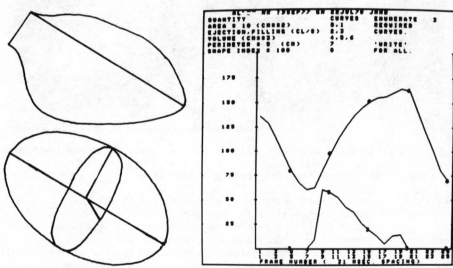

Fig. 9 Ellipsoidal model.

Fig. 10 Graphs of ventricular volume and its first derivative.

As already mentioned, the other category of information sought from
ventricular outlines is segmental outline motion analysis (Figure 11).
Analysis may include only the two frames of the sequence corresponding
to end-diastole and end-systole, or may include multiple frames. In
either case, the technique involves dividing each outline (represented
as before by a BOUNDARY) into a number of segments, though different
workers disagree as to the appropriate number to use. The motion of
each segment (which can be represented by a POINT or an ARC) is then
described by tables or graphs, or, in the case of multiple frame
analysis, by relief maps (Gibson and Brown 1976).

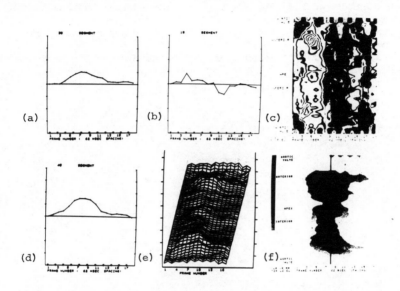

Fig.   11 Segmental outline motion analysis.
       (a),(b) Displacement with respect to their initial positions (as a
               function of time) of two selected segments.
       (c) Segmental velocity.
       (d) Displacements of 60 segments equally spaced along the outline.
       (e) Same information as (d), but represented by contour-line map.
       (f) Same information as (d),but represented by grey-level relief map

6. Summary

We have described the types of operation on images that are of general
usefulness in analysis of images. By developing standard Pascal software
incorporating predefined data structures and procedures for image
analysis, we have achieved considerable flexibility in selecting
algorithms while reducing the effort required to create applications
packages (in this case, for angiography). We have illustrated how current
technology permits the implementation of an analysis system with a
completely programmable architecture that is especially designed for
efficient execution of this image analysis software. The availability
of this type of system may encourage more widespread use of analysis
techniques that until now have been restricted to relatively few centres
because of their difficulty and expense of implementation.

Acknowledgment

We thank Dr D J Rowlands for supplying cineangiograms for our development work.

References

Barrett W A, Clayton P D and Warner H R 1980 Comput. Biomed. Res. 13 522

Brunt J N H, Taylor C J and Rowlands D J 1979 Computers in Cardiology ed K L Ripley and H G Ostrow (Long Beach: IEEE Computer Society) pp 437-40

Gibson D G and Brown D J 1976 7th L H Gray Conference: Medical Images (London: Institute of Physics) pp 323-35

Jensen K and Wirth N 1975 Pascal: User Manual and Report (New York: Springer-Verlag)

Slager C J, Reiber J H C, Schuurbiers J C H and Meester G T 1978 Comput. Biomed. Res. 11 491

Automated Quantification of Left Ventricular Angiograms

C J Slager, T E H Hooghoudt, P W Serruys, J H C Reiber and
J C H Schuurbiers

Thoraxcenter, Erasmus University and Academic Hospital Rotterdam-Dykzigt
P.O.Box 1738, 3000 DR Rotterdam.

Abstract

A system is described for the automated quantitative analysis of left
ventricular contrast cineangiograms. The automated acquisition of
left ventricular contours is performed with a dedicated hardwired
system, the Contouromat. Studies in piglets have shown that the detected contours provide new information on endocardial wall motion
based on endocardial landmark trajectories. The study of endocardial
landmark motion in 23 normal human individuals resulted in a new,
generally applicable method for the determination of regional ventricular wall motion. A clear distinction is made between locally observed wall motion and local wall performance. Examples of the application of the method in two different patient groups are described.

Introduction

The nature and extent of cardiac disease can be assessed accurately by
analysis of the left ventricular contrast cineangiogram. However, if this
analysis is based on visual interpretation, the results may be very
inconsistent as was demonstrated by Chaitman et al (1975) and Zir et al
(1976). For this reason and also because a more quantitative approach is
preferred, automated systems have been developed to obtain objective and
reproducible data from the angiogram (Robb et al 1971, Chow et al 1972,
Marcus et al 1972, Smalling et al 1976, Slager et al 1978, Bove et al
1978). The automated quantification of left ventricular volume was one of
the first applications of these systems. Initially, many volume calculating
methods have been described, but only few acquired general acceptance. The
area-length method introduced by Dodge (1960) and Sandler (1968) is widely
used as well as the method described by Chapman et al (1958). The volume
derived parameters are useful parameters of global cardiac function,
however, in these measurements, regional dysfunction may be masked by compen-
satory action of healthy wall segments. They have therefore very limited
value in the assessment of ischemic heart disease secondary to coronary
artery disorders. For this reason, several methods have been proposed
(Herman et al 1967, Leighton et al 1974, Harris et al 1974, Rickards et al
1977 and Chaitman et al 1973) to measure regional contractile function in
specific areas of the ventricle by analysis of the contrast angiogram.
However, these methods may introduce considerable error both in the
extent and in the direction of wall motion as was demonstrated by Ingels
et al (1980). For the accurate assessment of regional endocardial

wall function a new wall motion model has been developed which relies on the actual trajectories of anatomical structures (Slager et al 1979). The present study describes some results of such endocardial motion in 23 normal human hearts, in the heart of a patient without coronary artery disease before and after intracoronary administration of nifedipine* and in a patient with acute myocardial infarction in whom deobstruction of the coronary artery was successfully performed with streptokinase**. The present study was undertaken to demonstrate that this quantitative approach indeed provides new information on left ventricular function which is otherwise not available.

Left ventriculography

Ventriculography was performed in the 30° right anterior oblique (RAO) projection with 0.75 ml/kg Urographin 76*** at a flow rate of 18 ml/sec. Films were recorded with a 35 mm film camera at a rate of 50 frames/sec. When successive angiograms were made, care was taken to maintain the patient's position constant in relation to the X-ray equipment. Diaphragm motion was reduced by shallow inspiration avoiding the Valsalva manoeuvre The cardiac cycle with maximum contrast of the left ventricle - excluding extrasystolic and postextrasystolic beats - was chosen for analysis.

Automated acquisition of ventricular contours

The cineangiograms are converted into video format with a standard interlacing video camera (50Hz, 625 lines). The cineprojector is rotated such that the long axis of the left ventricle is about perpendicular to the horizontal scanning direction of the video system. With this optimized orientation there will never be more than two contour points on a videoline.

Automated contour detection is based upon a refined thresholding technique which uses an analog comparator to compare the video signal with the reference level. As soon as the video signal crosses the reference level, the comparator changes state, indicating the presence of a border point. The reference level is determined by the following factors:

-The local brightness levels of structures surrounding the border to be detected, assessed on a line to line basis.

-The "expectation window"; a narrow window which adapts dynamically to the ventricular shape. The center of this window is defined as having the same x-coordinate as the last detected border point on the previous video line. The comparator is enabled during the expectation window period only. During this period the calculated reference level is assigned a probability function such that the center of the window has the highest probability of being the next border point.

-The endocardial border in the previous detected frame. Since the border position changes little from frame to frame, the margin in the current frame can be approximated to a first degree with the margin of the previous frame. During contour detection the stored border positions are used to assign a probability function to the reference level.

-The endocardial border in the previous detected video field, which also assigns a probability function to the reference level. Since this information is updated at video field rate this factor introduces a kind of two dimensional filtering. This greatly reduces the influence of video noise.

* Bayer A.G., Wuppertal, F.R.G.
** Behring A.G., Marburg, F.R.G.
***Schering A.G., Berlin, Bergkammen, F.R.G.

The great advantage of this complex way of contour detection as realized in the Contouromat is that the detection process is rather insensitive to shading, nonhomogeneous mixing of the contrast agent in the left ventricle and overlapping of roentgen-opaque structures such as diaphragm, ribs and catheters, because the reference level is adjusted accordingly.

However, some problems still may occur, e.g. if extensive holes appear in the contrast distribution or if locally more than one border can be detected on the basis of calculated reference level. For example, this may be the case at the ventricular apex if an overshadowing rib has the same orientation as the ventricular border. In these cases a small writing tablet is used by the operator to move a cursor in the video image by means of which the detection process can be guided locally such that a correct contour is detected. The writing tablet is also used to indicate two starting points at both edges of the aortic valve in order to initiate the detection procedure in the first cineframe to be processed.

In figure 1a an example is given of a left ventricular angiogram as seen in the RAO projection, with the orientation as required by the contour detector. In figure 1b the same angiogram is shown with superimposition of the contour detected by the Contouromat.

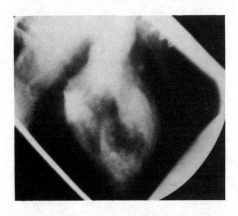 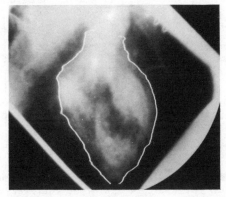

Figure 1a. Rotated contrast left ventriculogram as observed in the 30° RAO projection.

Figure 1b. Same angiogram with superimposition of the contour detected by the Contouromat.

When analyzing a sequence of cineframes the operator judges each detected contour of the Contouromat and makes corrections if necessary. As a result no significant discrepancies occur between the detected contours and manually drawn contours.

The contour acquisition time is determined almost completely by the time which is needed by the operator for inspection and correction of the contours. The Contouromat operates at video field rate, so that the contour detection itself takes much less than one second. In a previous study (Reiber et al 1978) the mean contour acquisition time has been measured by analysis of all frames over one or two cardiac cycles in a series of 29 consecutive angiograms. For those frames which required no correction the operator needed on the average 3.5 seconds to inspect the contour. Each additional correction required on the average 6 seconds. The percentage of frames which required one or more corrections was 45%. This resulted in a mean acquisition time of 12 sec per frame.

The"analog" contours produced by the Contouromat are digitized on a matrix of 256X384 points. By using a linear predictive coding technique each con- tour is represented completely by a total of only 256 bytes. The coded data are sent through a serial interface to a PDP 11/44 minicomputer, which stores the contours on a digital disk for subsequent processing.

Volume calculation

Following Chapman's method by assuming that the ventricular lumen is built up by a stack of circular slices, one slice for each videoline, the ven- tricular volume is calculated. Calibration is performed on the basis of the known dimensions of a cm-grid or a 100ml sphere. These objects are filmed following the ventriculographic procedure in the same position with respect to the X-ray system as the patient's left ventricle during the examination. The volumes thus obtained are further corrected for the angiographic over- estimation by the following regression equation (Heintzen et al 1974)

$$V_{true} = 0.72V_{measured} - 4.7 \text{ ml}$$

and indexed for body surface area. In figure 2 a graphical display of in- stantaneous volume and its time derivative is depicted as it is generated

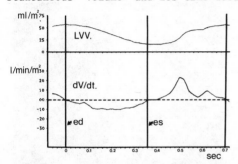

by the computer. Especially in the volume - time derivative plot small details can be recognized which illustrate how consistently the contours have been determined. The small relative maximum at 0.08 sec following the end-diastolic (ed) moment coincides with the opening of the aortic valve and can be recognized in all patients without valvular disease. Also, two filling phases can be observed; first, the rapid filling phase starting at 0.42 sec following ed and secondly, starting at 0.6 sec following ed, the contribution of the left atri- um. After generation of the volume plot, other well known parameters

Figure 2. Graphic display of ventricu- lar volume and its time derivative both indexed for body surface area. ed = end-diastole, es = endsystole.

e.g. ejection fraction, stroke volume and total cardiac output are calculated by the computer and displayed on a video monitor.

Endocardial wall motion

The high resolution outlining procedure of the Contouromat revealed small landmarks along the left ventricular contrast border, which can be followed throughout the cardiac cycle. The hypothesis that these landmarks actually represent specific anatomical sites has been tested by shooting minute "harpoons" in the endocardium in piglets by means of a specially construc- ted catheter. By comparing the systolic pathways of the naturally occurring landmarks with those of the "harpoons" their value could be substantiated. Although the landmark pathways appear at random sites along the ventricular border, mean pathways can be determined at other sites by interpolation between adjacent pathways. Following this approach, landmark pathways have been determined at 20 well defined sites along the end-diastolic contour, ten sites at the posterior wall distributed from the mitral valve fornix to the apex and also 10 sites at the anterior wall from base to apex.

In figure 3 an example of the systolic
pathways of the 20 endocardial landmarks in an individual animal is shown,
before marker insertion, as well as the
systolic pathways of the 5 metal markers implanted in the same ventricle.
The relation between the directions of
the endocardial landmark pathways and
the metal marker pathways was evaluated
by means of linear regression analysis.
For a total of 33 pathways in 8 piglets
a correlation coefficient of 0.86 was
found and a standard error of the
estimate of 10.3% In this comparison
the apical segments were excluded as

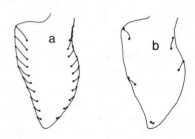

Figure 3. Systolic pathways of
endocardial landmarks (a) and
implanted markers (b) in a piglet.

the displacement of these segments is characterized by such short trajectories that accurate assessment of the direction of the pathways is almost
impossible. In general the anatomical landmark pathways tended to be longer
than the metal marker pathways by 10 to 20 %. This was caused mainly by an
increased transverse motion of the ventricular walls as was indicated by
the endocardial landmarks. A reason for this is that the contrast medium is
squeezed out of the intertrabecular spaces, a phenomenon that has been
observed also by many other investigators (e.g. Hugenholtz et al 1969,
McDonald 1970). In the RAO projection this squeezing effect is observed
particularly at the ventricular apex. As a result many investigators came
to the erroneous conclusion that the apex moves considerably towards the
base during systole (Leighton et al 1974, Rickards et al 1977) thereby
overestimating long axis shortening (Brower and Meester 1976, Rickards et
al 1977). In addition, contrast angiograms observed in the RAO projection
suggest a substantial rotation of the apex along the left ventricular long
axis, a phenomenon which is partially due to extrusion of dye by the
posterior papillary muscle. Earlier studies with epicardial and endocardial
markers had shown unmistakenly that the apex is remarkably stationary
during systole (Rushmer et al 1953, McDonald 1970, Hamilton and Rompf
1932). In keeping with these observations we found that the mean systolic
motion of the apical metal markers was less than a millimeter, although the
contrast angiogram in many instances would suggest considerable apical
upward motion and rotation, as is evident from inspection of figure 4.

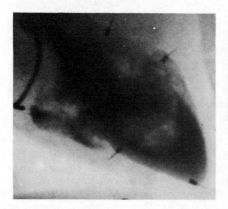
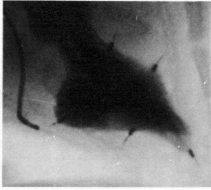

Figure 4. The end-diastolic (left) and end-systolic (right) frames of a pig
left ventriculogram with metal markers implanted in the endocardium.

Based on this evidence, models for the quantitative analysis of angiograms, particularly those proposed for the assessment of endocardial wall motion, should take into account these observations.

To obtain data of the motion of the human left ventricular endocardial wall, the systolic landmark pathways were analyzed in a series of 23 normal left ventriculograms. The results of this study are shown in figure 5. The indicated rectangular coordinate system is constructed in such a way that after the determination of the site at the anterior base (defined such that it has the same distance to the apex as the site at the mitral valve fornix), both sites at the base have equal y-coordinates. The other sites are distributed over the ventricular border in such a way that the lines connecting corresponding opposite sites (1-11, 2-12 etc.) divide the ventricular lumen into ten slices with equal heights. The mean systolic pathways are approximated by line vectors. The rectangles at the end of these pathways represent the standard deviations of the landmark positions at end-systole. The motion of the different sites from base to apex is characterized by a gradually decreasing y-componenent. The transverse motion as measured in the x-direction also decreases gradually from base towards apex. Furthermore, these data show that no single point exists that can be used as a center of motion. This conclusion seems to be in contradiction with the observations of Ingels et al (1978), who studied the motion of metal markers implanted in the midwall of human left ventricles. However, this method underestimates the transverse motion of the ventricular endocardial wall because the thickening of the part of the wall situated between the midwall marker and the endocardium is neglected.

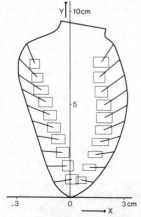

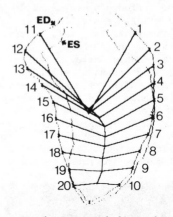

Figure 5. Systolic motion of the endocardial landmarks in 23 normal human left ventricles.

Figure 6. Computed directions of endocardial wall motion for an individual patient.

The analysis of anatomical landmarks thus has proven to be very useful. Tracing the landmark trajectories for each individual patient study is not practical, since that would require a fairly high quality angiogram and a considerable amount of analysis time. To circumvent these practical problems, a mathematical expression was formulated (Slager et al 1979), which makes the observed motion pattern applicable to the analysis of regional wall motion in other subjects. The computer uses this mathematical description to generate a pattern of expected motional directions for the individual sites defined at the end- diastolic contour, along which endocardial wall motion can be measured. In figure 6 the computer generated trajectories applied to an individual human left ventricle are shown.

Because the recognition of the apex and the mitral valve fornix from the detected end-diastolic contour is done automatically by the computer, no operator interaction is required for this part of the analysis.

In figure 7 the wall displacement data as a function of time are shown for an individual patient before (A) and after (B) intracoronary administration of a small bolus of nifedipine. Among other applications, nifedipine is increasingly employed by direct intracoronary injection in an effort to reverse spontaneously occurring or induced coronary spasm. In the left part of the figure segmental wall motion is depicted just before such an injection into the left main coronary artery. The arrows near the end-diastolic (ed) bar indicate the onset of displacement and the arrows near the moment of aortic valve closure (avc) indicate the moment of maximal displacement. A close correlation exists between the onset of displacement and the beginning of systole and also between the moment of maximum displacement and aortic valve closure. Only a small delay can be observed in the action of the posterior wall at sites 11-14. After the injection of nifedipine the dynamic behaviour of the ventricle changes dramatically for a short period of time. This situation is shown in the right part of figure 7. At the most affected sites (3-10 and 18-20) the onset of displacement is significantly delayed. After the moment of aortic valve closure, induced by the relaxation of the non-affected posterior wall sites, the anterior wall continues to move inwards, thus prolonging the isovolumic period.

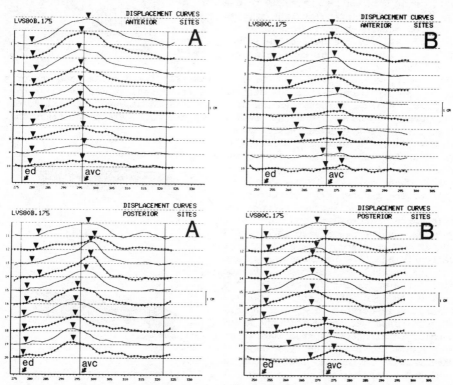

Figure 7. Effect of nifedipine into the left main coronary artery on left ventricular wall motion. Arrows indicate onset and the moment of maximal segmental wall displacement. ed= end-diastole, avc= aortic valve closure. A: control left ventriculogram. B: post-nifedipine ventriculogram.

Regional wall performance

A clear distinction has to be made between the locally observed wall motion at a particular ventricular site and the performance of the ventricular wall at that site. Even when extra-cardiac motion is excluded, the local wall performance cannot be deduced directly from the observed local motion in a simple way. When looking for example at the dynamic behaviour of the valvular plane, the observed motion in this region is almost the largest of all regions. However, the active contribution of these structures to the emptying of the ventricular lumen will be minimal. Apparently, the motion of the base towards the apex is the result of the longitudinal shortening of the ventricular wall as a whole. The same is true for the observed motion in this direction at all other sites of the ventricular wall. For this reason, new local ejection parameters were developed which have more functional significance than the local displacement or velocity.

Figure 8 depicts how the local displacement vector d can be decomposed in its x-and y-components. At each site of the ventricular end-diastolic contour a half-slice volume is defined with a radius equal to the radius of the ventricular lumen at that site and with a height equal to one tenth of the ventricular long axis as measured between base and apex. At the end of systole the half-slice volume at each site is calculated again from the local displacement vector d_x. Because the reduced height of the slice at end-systole cannot be derived with sufficient accuracy from the displacement data, a fixed shortening fraction of 14% is used, based on our observations in normal individuals. The contribution of this factor to the reduction of the slice volume is very small when compared to the contribution of the reduced slice diameter. As a next step local stroke volumes are calculated. Normalization of these volumes to the associated local half end-diastolic slice volumes gives the regional ejection fraction (REF) and to the global end-diastolic volume gives the so called contribution of a region to global ejection fraction (CREF), respectively. The sum of all 20 CREF data at the different sites equals global ejection fraction.

In figure 9 the percentile range of REF values in normal individuals is depicted. The median of the regional ejection fraction at the sites near the ventricular base is 50 to 60%, which is the smallest of all values. At the ventricular apex the median reaches a maximum of about 90%.

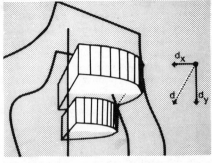

Figure 8. The displacement vector d is decomposed in its x- and y-components to measure regional stroke volumes and ejection fractions.

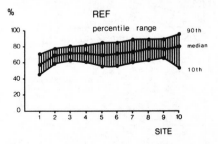

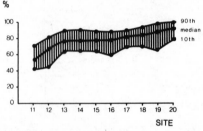

Figure 9. Percentile range of regional ejection fraction (REF) in normal individuals.

The REF parameter is particularly useful to study the local performance of the ventricular wall because of the narrow percentile range of normal values and its ease of interpretation being similar to the well known global ejection fraction.

The CREF parameter gives better insight into the relative importance of the different regions with respect to their contribution to global ventricular function. In figure 10 an example is given of a CREF determination from the angiogram of a patient treated with the thrombolytic agent streptokinase during the acute stage of anterior myocardial infarction. The end-diastolic and end-systolic left ventricular contours of the same patient were shown in figure 6. The solid line connects the individual CREF data. The dashed line represents the situation 3 weeks after the successful recanalization. Although the normal values as measured in the study group of normal individuals (dashed area) are not reached, ventricular function has improved not only at the anterior but also at the inferior wall sites. This finding that not only the infarct related area improves after the successful treatment with streptokinase but also the non-affected wall area has been measured consistently in a study group of five patients with anterior myocardial infarction and in a study group of six patients with inferior myocardial infarction.

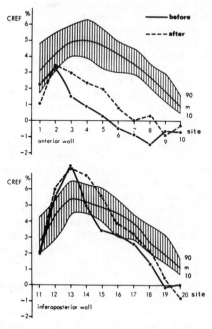

Figure 10. Contribution of different regions to global ejection fraction (CREF) before and after treatment with streptokinase in an individual patient.

Conclusion

Automated detection of left ventricular contours from the contrast cineangiogram, with the subsequent quantification of derived geometric parameters, allows a detailed analysis of global and regional left ventricular function which results in an improved diagnostic accuracy. This is not only useful for routine clinical work but essential for the accurate evaluation of therapeutic interventions.

References

Bove A.A., Kreulen T.H., Spann J.F.: Computer analysis of left ventricular dynamic geometry in man. Am. J. Cardiol. 41: 1239, 1978.

Brower R.W. and Meester G.T.: Computer based methods for quantifying regional left ventricular wall motion from cine ventriculograms. Comp. in Cardiol. 3: 55–62, IEEE Comp. Soc., Long Beach, California, 1976.

Chaitman B.R., Bristow J.D., Rahimtoola S.H.: Left ventricular wall motion assessed by using fixed external reference systems. Circ. 48:1043, 1973.

Chaitman B.R., DeMots H., Bristow J.D., Roesch J., Rahimtoola S.H.: Objective and subjective analysis of left ventricular angiograms, Circ. 52: 420, 1975.

Chapman C.B., Baker O., Reynolds J., Bonte F.J.: Use of biplane cinefluo-rography for measurement of ventricular volume. Circ. 18:1105-1117, 1958.

Chow C.K., Kaneko T.: Automatic boundary detection of the left ventricle from cineangiograms. Comput. Biom. Res. 5: 388, 1972.

Dodge H.T., Sandler H., Ballew D.W., Lord J.D. Jr.: The use of biplane angiocardiography for measurement of left ventricular volume in man. Am. Heart J. 60: 762, 1960.

Hamilton W.F., Rompf J.H.: Movements of the base of the ventricle and the relative consistancy of the cardiac volume. Amer. J. Physiol. 102: 559-565, 1932.

Harris L.D., Clayton P.D., Marshall H.W., Warnet H.R.: A technique for the detection of asynergistic motion in the left ventricle. Comp. Biomed. Res. 7: 380, 1974.

Heintzen P.H., Brenneke R., Bürsch J.H., Lange P., Malerczyk V., Moldenhauer K., Onnasch D.: Automated Video-Angiographic Image Analysis. Comp. in Card. 1: 67-75, IEEE Comp. Soc., Long Beach, Calif., 1974.

Herman M.V., Heinle R.A., Klein M.D., Gorlin R.: Localized disorders in myocardial contraction. N. Eng. J. Med. 227: 222, 1967.

Hugenholtz P.G., Kaplan E., Hill E.: Determination of left ventricular wall thickness by angiocardiography. Amer. Heart J. 78: 513, 1969.

Ingels N.B., Mead C.W., Daughters G.T., Stinson E.B. and Alderman E.L.: A new method for assessment of left ventricular wall motion. Comp. in Card. 5: 57-61, IEEE Comp. Soc., Long Beach, California, 1978.

Ingels N.B., Jr., Daughters G.T., Stinson E.B., Alderman E.L.: Evaluation of methods for quantitating left ventricular segmental wall motion in man using myocardial markers as standard. Circ. 61: 966 - 972, 1980.

Leighton R.F., Wilt S.M., Lewis R.P.: Detection of hypokinesis by a quanti-tative analysis of left ventricular cineangiograms. Circ. 50:121, 1974.

Marcus M.L., Schuette W.H., Whitehouse W.C., Bailey J.J., Glancy D.L.: An automated method for measurement of ventricular volume. Circ.45:65, 1972.

McDonald I.G.: The shape and movements of the human left ventricle during systole. Am. J. Cardiol. 26: 221, 1970.

Reiber J.H.C., Slager C.J., Schuurbiers J.C.H., Meester G.T.: Contouromat: A hard-wired left ventricular angio processing system. II. Performance evaluation. Comput. Biomed. Res. 11: 503 - 523, 1978.

Rickards A., Seabra-Gomes R., Thurstone P.: The assessment of regional abnormalities of the left ventricle by angiography. Eur. J. Cardiol. 5, 167, 1977.

Robb R.A., Computer-aided contour determination and dynamic display of individual cardiac chambers from digitized serial angiocardiographic films. Ed. by Heintzen P.H., G. Thieme Publishers pg. 170, 1971.

Rushmer R.F., Crystal D.K., Wagner C.: The functional anatomy of ventricular contraction. Circ. Res. 1: 162-170, 1953.

Sandler H., Dodge H.T., The use of single plane angiocardiograms for the calculation of left ventricular volume in man. Am. Heart J. 75:325, 1968.

Slager C.J., Reiber J.H.C., Schuurbiers J.C.H. and Meester G.T.: Contouromat: A hardwired left ventricular angioprocessing system. I. Design and application. Comp. Biomed. Res. 11: 491-502, 1978.

Slager C.J., Hooghoudt T.E.H., Reiber J.H.C., Schuurbiers J.C.H., Booman F. and Meester G.T.: Left ventricular contour segmentation from anatomical landmark trajectories and its application to wall motion analysis. Comp.in Card. 6 : 347-350, IEEE Comp. Soc., Long Beach, Calif., 1979.

Smalling R.W., Skolnick M.H., Myers D., Shabetai R., Cole J.C., Johnston D. Digital boundary detection, volumetric and wall motion analysis of left ventricular cineangiograms. Comput. Biol. Med. 6: 73, 1976.

Zir L.M., Miller S.W., Dinsmore R.E., Gilbert J.P., Harthorne J.W.: Interobserver variability in coronary angiography. Circ. 53: 627, 1976.

Computer-Aided Analysis of Coronary Obstructions from Monoplane Cineangiograms and Three-Dimensional Reconstruction of an Arterial Segment from Two Orthogonal Views

JHC Reiber, JJ Gerbrands*, CJ Kooijman, GJ Troost*, JCH Schuurbiers, CJ Slager, A den Boer, PW Serruys

Laboratory for Clinical and Experimental Image Processing, Thoraxcenter, Erasmus University, P.O. Box 1738, 3000 DR Rotterdam, The Netherlands

*Information Theory Group, Delft University of Technology, P.O. Box 5031, 2600 GA Delft, The Netherlands

Abstract

The computer-aided analysis of coronary obstructions from cineangiograms is described. First, the assessment of the percentage diameter reduction from single view angiograms is discussed. This method requires the delineation of the contours of the artery and the analysis of the diameter function. Next, a method is described to transform the brightness values in the digital image into calibrated absorption profiles, thus creating the possibility to assess percentage area reduction from single views. Finally, the three-dimensional reconstruction of an arterial segment from two orthogonal views is discussed.

Introduction

To visualize the morphology of the coronary arterial tree X-ray coronary angiograms are obtained in a cardiac catheterization laboratory after selective injection of an X-ray contrast agent into one of the main coronary arteries. The images are recorded on 35 mm cinefilm with a cine-camera mounted on top of the image intensifier of the X-ray system; the film speed usually is taken between 25 and 50 frames/s. The film provides the clinician with detailed information about the morphology of the coronary arterial tree, thus creating the possibility to investigate the presence, the severity and the functional significance of coronary obstructions.

However, the diagnostic value of coronary angiograms is severely limited by the usual visual and therefore subjective interpretation of the images. Inter- and intra-observer variations from 8 to 37% in judging the location and severity of coronary obstructions from visual interpretations have been well documented in the literature (Detre et al 1975, Zir et al 1976, De Rouen et al 1977). Also, from visual interpretation it is very difficult to accurately assess the hemodynamic effect of a narrowing in a coronary artery or bypass graft, since this requires accurate knowledge about the shape and absolute size of the obstruction. Moreover, the effects of short-term interventions (such as transluminal coronary angioplasty and medical therapy), as well as long-term interventions (as surgical therapy) cannot be evaluated as accurately as would be desirable.

Due to the limited value that can be attached to diagnoses based on the visual interpretation of the images only coarse classifications can be used to distinguish patient groups and for coronary research studies, particularly cooperative studies.

In view of the clinical need for optimal interpretation of these images, it is attractive to develop an objective and reproducible quantitation method. Such a method should eliminate the imperfections mentioned above as much as possible and particularly be suitable for accurate classification of patients for coronary bypass surgery. Further developments of such a system could possibly lead to the implementation of a coronary database system. The main incentives for the design of such a system are: 1) the need for reproducible and standardized reading and scoring of coronary angiograms, and 2) the possibility of computer storage and retrieval of these data with fast and accurate access for the benefit of scientific and clinical research.

This paper describes procedures that have been developed for the computer-aided quantitative analysis of selected coronary lesions. These procedures have been implemented at the Laboratory for Clinical and Experimental Image Processing of the Thoraxcenter in Rotterdam in close cooperation with the Information Theory Group of Delft University of Technology.

After a brief overview of the pertinent literature on quantitative coronary angiography, the implemented Coronary Angiography Analysis System (CAAS) will be discussed. The first quantitation procedure to be described deals with the assessment of the percentage diameter reduction of a coronary obstruction from single view angiograms. This method requires the accurate delineation of the contours of the coronary artery at the selected obstruction. From these contours the diameter function is obtained. The percentage diameter reduction as well as the extent of the obstruction are computed from the diameter function. However, it will be shown that percentage diameter reduction in a single view is of limited diagnostic value. To obtain the more relevant cross-sectional percentage area reduction, a densitometric procedure has been developed which uses the brightness information within the artery. Finally, we will discuss the feasibility to extend the densitometric procedure to the three-dimensional reconstruction of a coronary segment from two orthogonal views.

Overview of pertinent literature

Over the last ten years various systems for the quantitation of the coronary arteries have been described in the literature. To manually measure absolute sizes of coronary arterial segments at a number of discrete positions cross-hair measuring systems and vernier calipers have been used (Gensini et al 1971, Rafflenbeul et al 1976). A semi-automated computerized method for the analysis of biplane coronary cineangiograms has been described by Bolson et al (1977) and Brown et al (1977). This system requires manual tracing of the coronary lesions in two projected angiographic views. The contour data are transmitted to a digital computer. The two views are matched and a 3-dimensional representation of the vessel is reconstructed assuming elliptical lumen allowing the computation of various clinically significant parameters. A semi-automated computer-aided densitometric procedure for the evaluation of stenotic lesions in coronary angiograms requiring extensive operator-interaction has been published by Sandor et al (1979). Pochon et al (1982) have also employed densitometric procedures in an attempt to derive cross-sectional area measures from single view coronary cineangiograms. Starmer and Smith (1974) were the first to report on extensive computer processing methods for coronary

angiograms (Smith and Starmer 1976). They developed algorithms for the
efficient measurement, representation and storage of coronary trees by
computer from biplane coronary arteriograms. Clinical results were not
published after their initial publications. A semi-automated computer-
based system was developed by Sanders et al (1979). The boundaries of the
artery are manually traced with a light pen. Subsequently, a computer
algorithm defines a more accurate delineation of the edges from video
converted cineangiograms. Selzer et al (1976, 1982) have developed computer algorithms for the automated contour detection of selected coronary
lesions. Required operator-interaction consists of indicating a number of
points along the approximate midline of the vessel with a sonic digitizer.
The contours of the segment are then detected automatically from video
converted digital data. Various luminal measures are computed from the
obtained contour data.

The Coronary Angiography Analysis System

The Coronary Angiography Analysis System (CAAS) is a PDP-11/44 interactive image processing system developed and implemented in our laboratory
(Booman et al 1979, Gerbrands et al 1980). A block diagram of the system
is given in Fig. 1.

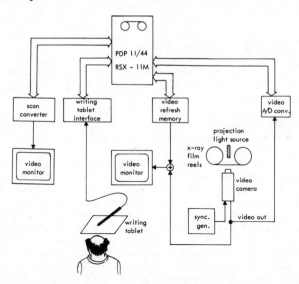

Fig. 1. Block diagram, Coronary Angiography Analysis System.

To analyze a selected cineframe, the film is placed on a cine-video
converter that has been developed in our laboratory in cooperation with
the Central Research Workshop of the Medical Faculty, Rotterdam. This cine-
video converter is a mobile unit consisting of a standard 35 mm Vanguard
cinefilm transport mechanism mounted on top of a cabinet (Fig. 2).
The image is projected downward into the cabinet onto the surface
of the 1.5" vidicon tube of a Sierra Scientific video camera via a drum
with 6 different lens systems, which allow the selection of the desired
optical magnification factor from $1/\sqrt{2}:1$ to $4:1$ in multiplicative steps
of $\sqrt{2}$. Magnification of $1:1$ is defined   such that the projected image
of a standard cineframe with dimensions 24x18 mm precisely fills the
scanning area of the video camera.

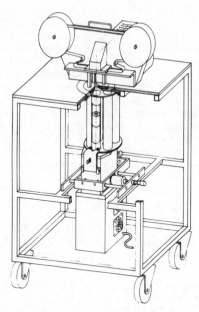

Fig. 2. Drawing of cine-video converter

The video camera is mounted on a movable x-y stage, so that any area of interest in the 35 mm cineframe can be selected with the appropriate magnification factor. The cinefilm transport, the selection of the desired optical magnification as well as the x-y positioning of the video camera are all operated through the PDP 11/44 host computer. The different functions in the converter are controlled by a built-in Intel 8085 microprocessor.

An external crystal-controlled video synchronization generator with a basic frequency of 14.4 MHz controls the video camera and the analog-to-digital converter in   Fig. 1. The video A/D-converter identifies 800 picture elements (pixels) per video line, and   both the even and odd lines of the 2:1 interlaced video system are utilized. The grey scale resolution of the digital data is 256 levels. A selected region in the video image is digitized column-by-column under program control and sent on DMA-basis through a DR 11-B interface to the host computer. To reduce the effects of electronic noise, the image may be digitized a number of times and averaged. The actual processing unit is the PDP 11/44 minicomputer with 128k words of memory running under the RSX-11M Operating System. The digital image can be visualized by writing the data onto the storage tube of a video scan-converter. Graphics and the contours of the analyzed arteries can be superimposed in the original video image with a video refresh memory organized as a 600x800 matrix with 1 bit information. Operator-interaction is possible with a writing-tablet.

Contour analysis

A simple measure to quantify the severity of a coronary obstruction is the percentage diameter reduction of the obstruction with respect to a reference region, with the diameter defined as the width of the artery perpendicular to its centerline. To compute this parameter the boundaries of the coronary arterial segment need to be determined. The procedure

developed for edge detection and diameter analysis will be described in
concise form, as it has been reported elsewhere (Booman et al 1979,
Gerbrands et al 1980). The processing of a selected coronary obstruction
is performed in a number of steps by using regions of interest of 96x96
pixels. The user indicates a number of center positions with the writing
tablet, such that the straight line segments connecting consecutive pairs
of these points are within the artery (Fig. 3a). These line segments form
the tentative centerline for the lesion. The first part of this centerline
is used to define the first 96x96 region to be digitized. After the contours within this region have been detected, the next region to be digitized is defined by the last centerline segment of the current region and
the next centerline segment. The overlap of consecutive regions is taken
such that connectivity of the contours is assured (Fig. 3b). Each region
is digitized twice and averaged for noise reduction. For the same reason,
the digital data are smoothed with an unweighted 3x3 operator prior to
detection of the edge points.

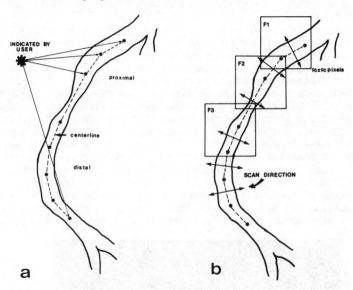

Fig. 3 (a) To analyze a selected coronary arterial segment the user
            indicates a number of center positions. The interpolated
            straight line segments form the tentative centerline.
       (b) The locations of the 96x96 digitization matrices are de-
            termined by the tentative centerline. The scan directions
            are defined perpendicular to the corresponding centerline
            segments.

For each part of the piece-wise linear tentative centerline, the direction perpendicular to that part is defined as the local search or scan
direction. The straight lines through the matrix in the scan direction are
called the scanlines. On a specific scanline, the two edge positions of
the artery are detected by applying a one-dimensional averaging first-
derivative operator to the brightness values. The possible positions of
the edge points on this scanline are restricted to expectation windows
defined by the two detected edge points on the previous scanline. At the
transitions of tentative centerline segments with different direction
coefficients, there are edge points missing at one side and clusters of

edge points at the other side. The missing points are obtained by interpolation, whereas a thinning operator is applied to the clusters.

After processing all 96x96 regions of interest, a least-squares
second-order polynomial fit is applied to each of the two edges yielding
the final contours.

From the contours the diameter function D(i) is determined by computing the shortest distances between the left and right contour positions.
From the minimum D_m of the diameter function and the mean diameter D_r
at a user-indicated reference position, the percentage diameter reduction
is computed as :

$$\text{D-STENOSIS} = \left(1 - \frac{D_m}{D_r}\right) \times 100\%$$

The mean diameter D_r is computed as the average of 11 diameter values in
a symmetric region with center at the indicated reference position. Furthermore, the extent of the obstruction is determined automatically from
the diameter function.

The final result of the procedure for an obstruction in the Obtuse
Marginal branch is illustrated in Fig. 4. The smoothed contours are superimposed on the original video image. Administrative data are plotted at
the top. The diameter function is shown at the right side of the image;
the calibrated diameter values in mm are plotted along the ordinate and
the centerline positions from the proximal to the distal part along the
abscissa. For this particular case the reference position was defined at
the left side of the obstructive lesion as indicated in the diameter
function by the extended vertical line. For this obstruction we find a
percentage diameter reduction of 50%. The extent of the stenotic lesion is
indicated in the diameter function by the two dotted lines and is represented by the shaded area superimposed on this artery. Usually, the reference position is also marked in the artery by a straight line connecting the opposing contour sides. However, in the example of   Fig. 4 the
reference position was defined at the boundary of the computed lesion and
as a result the reference marker is overwritten by the shaded obstructive
area.

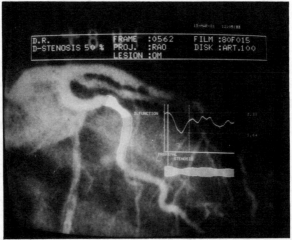

Fig. 4. Computer output of analyzed lesion in Obtuse Marginal branch.
A percentage diameter reduction of 50% with respect to the
user-defined reference region is found.

Calibration of the diameter data is achieved by using the intracardiac catheter as a scaling device. To this end, the contours of part of
the projected catheter are detected automatically in a way similar as
described above for the arterial segment. A mean diameter value is determined in pixels, so that the calibration factor can be computed from the
known size of the catheter. Particularly for intervention studies the
absolute dimensions of pre-, post- and stenotic segments are of great
clinical importance.

It is clear from the above that the computed percentage diameter
narrowing of an obstruction depends heavily on the selected reference
position. In arteries with a focal obstructive lesion and a clearly normal
proximal arterial segment, the choice of the reference region is straight-
forward and simple. However, in cases where the proximal part of the
arterial segment shows combinations of stenotic and ectatic areas, the
choice may be very difficult. To circumvent these problems as much as
possible, we have implemented an alternative method to express the
severity of a coronary obstruction, which is not dependent on a user-
defined reference region. First, the extent of the obstruction is
determined from the diameter function. Then, for both the proximal and the
distal segment, a reference diameter value is defined by the 90 percentile
of the corresponding diameter values. The diameter values of a possibly
present post-stenotic dilation are automatically excluded in these calculations. These two reference diameter values are then assumed to be a
measure for the normal size of the proximal and distal segments
respectively. Similarly, normal sizes over the obstructive lesion can be
obtained by interpolation between the proximal and distal reference
values. The resulting normal size of the arterial segment of Fig. 4 is
shown in Fig. 5, with the difference area between this boundary and the
detected contours marked, being a measure for the atherosclerotic plaque.
The interpolated percentage diameter-stenosis is then computed by
comparing the minimal diameter value at the obstruction with the
corresponding interpolated diameter value. For Fig. 5 an interpolated
diameter stenosis of 50% results. Further evaluation of this method is
necessary to determine its diagnostic value.

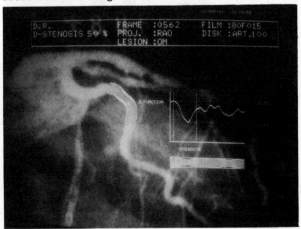

Fig. 5. For the lesions of Fig. 4 the normal size of the artery has
been estimated from the normal proximal and distal diameter
values(90-percentile). The marked area is a measure for the
atherosclerotic plaque. An interpolated percentage diameter
stenosis of 50% results.

The accuracy of the quantitation method has been validated with ten copper models of obstructed coronary arteries having circular cross sections. The percentage diameter narrowing for the set of models range from 0% to 90% in steps of approximately 10%. The proximal and distal diameters of the models equal 4.0 mm and all diameters are produced with an accuracy of 0.01 mm. Cinefilms were made of the models immersed in a water basin with 10 cm of water, with the same X-ray system settings as during coronary angiography. The cinefilms were analyzed as described above. The computer measurements in terms of D-STENOSIS were compared with the known true percentages in a linear regression analysis. The accuracy was found to be 1.9% and the precision 1.6%.

Densitometric procedure

Since the luminal cross section at a coronary obstruction is frequently irregular in shape, percentage diameter reduction measured in a single projection is of limited diagnostic value. The hemodynamic resistance of an obstruction is determined to a great extent by the changes in the cross-sectional areas of the lumen. Computation of the cross-sectional area reduction from the percentage diameter reduction measured in a single view requires the assumption of a circular cross section, an assumption which hardly ever holds. The resulting error may be reduced by incorporating two orthogonal projections and computing elliptical cross sections. However, with the often occurring eccentric lesions even this last approach provides poor results, as can be shown with the following example. Fig. 6 diagrammatically portrays and depicts the complex problems stemming from a slit-like stenosis having a crescent shape. In cases such as this, even three or more views will not "provide a faithful portrayal of their severity" (Gensini 1975). A lateral "view" of the crescent would suggest a 10% reduction in lumen diameter; a "left oblique" would yield a 25% narrowing and an "anteroposterior" would imply a 60% stenosis. Even a technique of quantitating area stenosis from two orthogonal measurements and computing area based on an elliptical model would fail to describe accurately the severity of this lesion.

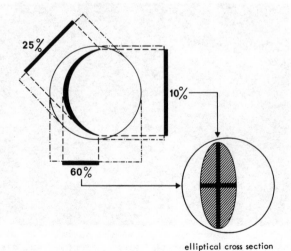

elliptical cross section

Fig. 6. Potential errors in the evaluation of the severity of a crescent-like lesion from single and orthogonal views.

However, some clue to the presence of this grossly asymmetrical lesion will exist, because the density of contrast medium is markedly reduced in that area, even though the caliber seems normal. Unexplained diminution of the opacity of a contrast-filled lumen (density changes) should alert the angiographer to the severity of the luminal narrowing. If one could constitute the relationship between the path length of the X-rays through the artery and the brightness values in the digital image, one would obtain the information required to compute the cross-sectional areas from a single view (Fig. 7).

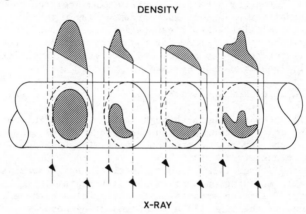

Fig. 7. Schematic illustration of the relationship between the irradiated object thickness and the density in the angiographic image.

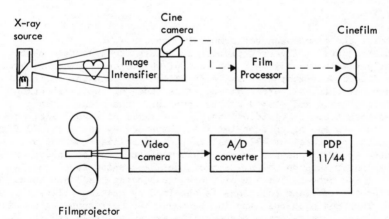

Fig. 8. Block diagram of X-ray/video imaging system.

The block diagram of the complete X-ray/video chain is given in Fig.8. Constitution of the relationship between path length and brightness values requires detailed analysis of the complete imaging system. In a simplified approach, we are only interested in the static properties of the system. Analysis of the static transfer function of each link in the chain reveals that computation of the complete transfer function is very difficult.There is a large number of parameters involved, many of which are spatially variant. For the time being, we have settled for the following compromise.

For the first part of the chain from the X-ray source to the output of the
image intensifier we use a simple model. From the output of the image intensifier up to the brightness values in the digital image we measure the
transfer function on a point-by-point basis. In this paper the basic principles of this technique will be described. A more extensive description
can be found in Reiber et al (1982a).

Let p_c denote a position in the plane of the digital image which
lies within the contours as detected following the method described in the
previous section, and let p_b denote a background position just outside
the contours.   Let $E(p_c)$ be the cinefilm exposure from the output of
the image intensifier at a position corresponding with position p_c in
the image plane; similarly $E(p_b)$ can be defined for the background position. Using Lambert-Beer's Law for the X-ray absorption and applying
certain models for the X-ray source and the image intensifier, the
following relationship can be derived :

$$d(p_c) = k_1 \cdot (\log E(p_b) - \log E(p_c)), \qquad (1)$$

where $d(p_c)$ is the path length through the contrast agent in the artery
at position p_c and k_1 a constant. In this simple model all parameters
of the source, the absorption process and the image intensifier are mapped
into the single unknown constant k_1.

The mapping T from film exposure levels to brightness values in the
digital image is measured on a point-by-point basis. This mapping T is determined in the following way. Prior to the cardiac catheterization the
first 10 frames of the cinefilm are exposed homogeneously with a sen-
sitometer having the same color temperature as the output screen of the
image intensifier. The calibration frames are exposed according to an
exponential function :

$$E(p) = k_2 \cdot 2^{-n} \qquad (2)$$

with n being the frame sequence number $(0 \leqslant n \leqslant 9)$.
Following the cardiac investigation these frames are processed photo-
graphically simultaneously with the rest of the coronary cineangiogram, so
that the film development process is identical for both the calibration
frames and the clinical coronary cineframes. Each of the calibration
frames is digitized and stored in the computer. Subsequently, each
digitized test frame is divided into 432 subimages of size 28x28; in each
subimage the average brightness level is computed. By using all 10 frames
this results in a total of 432 local mapping functions, each of which is
represented by its 10 sample points. Intermediate function values are obtained by linear interpolation. Each of the 432 mapping functions is
assigned to the center position of the corresponding 28x28 subimage. The
mapping for intermediate positions is obtained by spatial bilinear interpolation. Thus for each position in the image the corresponding mapping
function defines the relation between film exposure levels and the resulting digitized video levels.

The inverse T^{-1} of this mapping must exist to be able to compute the
exposures $E(p_c)$ and $E(p_b)$ from the video levels $V_d(p_c)$ and $V_d(p_b)$,
respectively in the digitized image. For position p_c we find

$$n(p_c) = T^{-1} \left[V_d(p_c), p_c \right] \qquad (3)$$

Because of the applied interpolations n may now take on any value between
0 and 9. Equations (2) and (3) yield :

$$\log E(p_c) = k_3 \cdot T^{-1} \left[V_d(p_c), p_c \right] + k_4 \qquad (4)$$

A similar equation can be defined for the background position p_b.

The brightness values $V_d(p_c)$ and $V_d(p_b)$, in the projected artery and the background, respectively, are now used to compute the length of the absorption path at position p_c by combining (1) and (4) into

$$d(p_c) = k_5 \cdot \{ T^{-1} \left[V_d(p_b), p_b) \right] - T^{-1} \left[V_d(p_c), p_c \right] \}, \qquad (5)$$

where k_5 is an unknown spatially independent constant. In this way the brightness values in the projected artery can be calibrated in terms of the amount of X-ray absorption. By means of this calibration procedure many nonlinear and spatially variant effects in the film processing and the film-video system are taken into account.

The percentage cross-sectional area reduction of a selected lesion is then obtained as follows. When selecting the cineframe for the densitometric analysis of a particular arterial segment, we make sure that the main axis of the segment in 3-D space is reasonably parallel to the projection plane. The contours of the artery are detected as described. On each scanline perpendicular to the centerline, a profile of brightness values is measured. This profile is transformed into an exposure profile by means of equation (4). The background contribution is estimated by computing the linear regression line through the background points directly left and right of the detected contours. Subtraction of this background portion from the absorption profile within the arterial contours according to equation (5) yields the net cross-sectional absorption profile. Integration of this function results in a measure for the cross-sectional area at the particular scanline. This procedure is illustrated in Fig. 9.

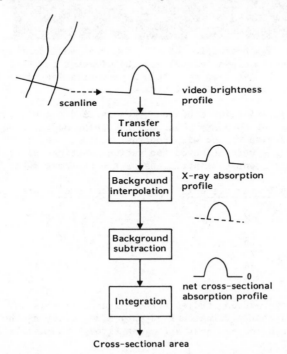

Fig. 9. Schematic drawing for determining the cross-sectional area data from the densitometric information within the arterial segment.

By repeating this procedure for all the scanlines,the cross-sectional area function A(i) is obtained. It is clear that a homogeneous mixing of the contrast agent with the blood must be assumed for the measurements to be correct. Fig. 10 shows the clinical case of Fig. 4 with the computed diameter function (upper curve) and area function (lower curve). The severity of the obstruction can now be expressed as a percentage area reduction, by comparing the minimal area value at the obstruction with the mean value at the selected reference position. For this particular obstruction we found a percentage area reduction of 81%. Assuming a model with circular cross sections, a percentage area reduction of 75% would have resulted, thus slightly underestimating the true severity of the obstruction.

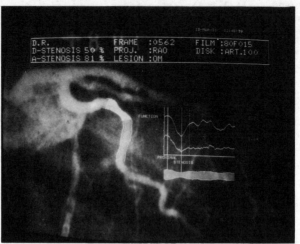

Fig. 10. For the obstruction of Fig. 4 the densitometric area
         function (lower curve) and the diameter function (upper
         curve) have been computed. A percentage densitometric area
         reduction of 81% is found.

A preliminary validation study has been carried out with cinefilms of four perspex models of coronary obstructions. These models have circular cross sections and were filled with contrast medium. The following area reduction percentages were measured for various settings of the X-ray system and with different concentrations of the contrast agent :

True %-area stenosis	Measured %-area stenosis		
	film 1	film 2	film 3
86	85	87	85
75	78	72	73
44	44	41	39
0	8	8	4

Extension of the evaluation studies to non-circular models and to post-mortem casts is currently being carried out. Also, studying the effects of dynamic flow of blood and contrast agent through the models is being anticipated.

3-D Reconstruction

If two orthogonal projections are available, the three-dimensional shape of the selected arterial segment can be reconstructed slice-by-slice in the following way. The two projections are analyzed sequentially in the way described, providing two densitometric absorption profiles for each cross section. From these two profiles and by exploiting the a priori information concerning the shape of a previously reconstructed adjacent slice, the cross-sectional shape is reconstructed by means of a minimum cost reconstruction algorithm. This method will be outlined below. Details may be found in Reiber et al (1982b).

Under the assumption of complete and homogeneous filling of the artery with contrast agent and of the X-rays to be parallel at the structure of interest, we adopt the following discrete model. A slice of the artery is represented by a binary matrix. The matrix elements are "1" for positions that lie within the arterial cross section, and "0" for positions outside of it. In this discrete model the two absorption profiles obtained from the cineangiograms represent the row and column sums of this matrix. Therefore, we state our problem of reconstructing one slice as the reconstruction of a binary matrix from its row and column sums.

From combinatorial mathematics the conditions are known for the existence of no, one or more than one solution of this problem. In the ideal case without noise and measurement errors, there are many solutions, and other information has to be used to reduce the ambiguity. On physiological grounds, there must be a strong resemblance between two adjacent cross sections of the artery. We therefore reformulate our problem as the search for a binary matrix satisfying the projections with maximum resemblance to the previously reconstructed adjacent slice. It is attractive to incorporate a resemblance criterion in the reconstruction process directly, which we have achieved by introducing a cost coefficient $c(i,j)$ for every element (i,j) of the matrix, which represents the penalty for assigning that element the value "1" in the reconstruction. A simple example is to set $c(i,j)$ equal to zero if the matrix element (i,j) was an element of the arterial cross section in the previously reconstructed slice and equal to one otherwise. The minimum cost solution of the reconstruction problem will then show a high degree of similarity to the previous cross section.

Let $x(i,j)$ denote the (i,j)-element of the matrix to be reconstructed, $c(i,j)$ the corresponding cost coefficient, $\alpha(i)$ the sum of row i of the matrix and $\beta(j)$ the sum of column j. We formulate the following optimization process :

$$\text{Minimize } \sum_i \sum_j c(i,j) \cdot x(i,j) \tag{6}$$

under the constraints

$$\sum_j x(i,j) = \alpha(i) \qquad \forall\ i \tag{7}$$

$$\sum_i x(i,j) = \beta(j) \qquad \forall\ j \tag{8}$$

$$x(i,j) \in \{0,1\} \qquad \forall\ i,j \tag{9}$$

This optimization problem is related to the transportation problem in the Operations Research literature. It can be approached conveniently as a flow problem in a directed network.   Fig. 11 illustrates the correspondence between the matrix reconstruction problem and the network flow problem.

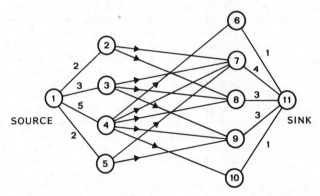

	1	4	3	3	1
2	0	1	1	0	0
3	0	1	1	1	0
5	1	1	1	1	1
2	0	1	0	1	0

Fig. 11. The matrix reconstruction problem and the network flow approach.

The capacities of the arcs directed away from the source are set equal to the row sums. The capacities of the arcs directed towards the sink are set equal to the column sums. The capacities of the intermediate arcs are set equal to unity. The actual flows of the intermediate arcs (either zero or one) correspond with the entries of the matrix of the reconstruction problem. The flow through the network is maximal, if the actual flows through the source and the sink arcs are equal to their capacities. For simplicity, only those intermediate arcs that do transport a unit of flow are given in Fig. 11. With each intermediate arc we associate the cost coefficient of the corresponding matrix element. We can then adapt algorithms from the Operations Research literature to find the minimum cost solution at maximal flow through the capacitated network.

This approach to the binary reconstruction problem from two ortho-gonal projections was originally developed by Slump and Gerbrands (1981) for the reconstruction of the left ventricle from biplane left ventricular angiograms. Since the two applications are basically identical, the algorithms actually implemented for the coronary arteries are very similar to those proposed for the reconstruction of the left ventricle.

Under practical circumstances, the acquired absorption profile data will be disturbed by noise and measurement errors and no single solution can be found, in general. The effects of these deviations on the recon-struction process are discussed in Reiber et al (1982b).

The two orthogonal frames required for the reconstruction are selected manually and the analyzed arterial segments in the two projections are aligned interactively by indicating two corresponding landmarks in the two frames. By this procedure the scales of both projections are matched as well. The first slice to be reconstructed is at the user-indicated reference region where the cross section of the artery is assumed to be elliptical in shape. A plot of an obstructed coronary arterial segment, reconstructed slice-by-slice from two orthogonal arteriograms, is given in Fig. 12. Notice that similar plots can be displayed for any viewing angle, independent of the original projection angles. For this particular example a total of 155 slices were reconstructed.

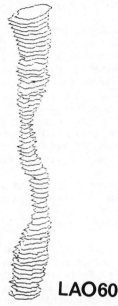

LAO60

Fig. 12. Three-dimensional representation of obstructed arterial segment reconstructed from two orthogonal projections.

Concluding Remarks

The diameter analysis procedure has been evaluated extensively and is clinically used as a diagnostic tool. Also, different studies on the effects of interventions on coronary morphology, such as drug administration during the cardiac catheterization and the percutaneous transluminal coronary angioplasty procedure (PTCA) have been or are being carried out (Serruys et al 1980). The densitometric area reduction analysis procedure has been applied to the PTCA-films. The first results from these clinical evaluations are certainly very promising (Serruys et al 1982). The 3-D reconstruction of coronary obstructions has not yet emerged from the research state. This technique is clinically of great importance since it may allow the computation of blood flow profiles and of the hemodynamic resistance of an obstruction.

Acknowledgments

This work has been supported in part by the Dutch Heart foundation under grant no's 77.084, 79.109 and 80.129. The authors wish to thank Mrs A Wagenaar for her secretarial assistance with the preparation of this manuscript.

References

Bolson E L, Brown B G, Dodge H T and Frimer M 1977 Proc. Digital
Equipment Computer Users Society pp 453-8
Booman F, Reiber J H C, Gerbrands J J, Slager C J, Schuurbiers J C H and
Meester G T 1979 Proc. Comp in Card pp 177-81
Brown B G, Bolson E, Frimer M and Dodge H T 1977 Circ 55 pp 329-37
De Rouen T A, Murray J A and Owen W 1977 Circ 55 pp 324-8
Detre K M, Wright E, Murphy M L and Takaro T 1975 Circ 52 pp 979-86
Gensini G G, Kelly A E, Da Costa B C B and Huntington P P 1971 Chest 60
pp 522-30
Gensini G G 1975 Coronary Angiography (London: Futura)
Gerbrands J J, Reiber J H C and Booman F 1980 Pattern Recognition in
Practice (Amsterdam: North Holland) pp 223-33
Pochon Y, Doriot P A, Rasoamanambelo L and Rutishauser W 1982
Angiography, Current Status and Future Developments (Berlin: Springer)
(in press)
Rafflenbeul W, Heim R, Dzuiba M, Henkel B and Lichtlen P 1976 Coronary
Angiography and Angina Pectoris (Stuttgart: Thieme) pp 255-65
Reiber J H C, Slager C J, Schuurbiers J C H, den Boer A, Gerbrands J J,
Troost G J, Scholts B, Kooijman C J and Serruys P W 1982a Digital Video
Image Techniques in Cardiovascular Radiology (Stuttgart: Thieme)(in
press)
Reiber J H C, Gerbrands J J, Troost G J, Kooijman C J and Slump C H 1982b
Digital Video Image Techniques in Cardiovascular Radiology (Stuttgart:
Thieme) (in press)
Sanders W J, Alderman E L and Harrison D C 1979 Proc. Comp in Card pp
15-20
Sandor T, Als A V and Paulin S 1979 Cath and Cardiovasc Diagn 5 pp 229-45
Selzer R H, Blankenhorn D H, Crawford D W, Brooks S H and Barndt R 1976
Proc. Caltech/JPL Conf on Image Processing Technology, Data Sources and
Software for Commercial and Scientific Applications pp 1-20
Selzer R H 1982 Proc. Workshop on Quantitative Evaluation of
Atherosclerosis (Springer) (in press)
Serruys P W, Steward R, Booman F, Michels R, Reiber J H C and Hugenholtz
P G 1980 Eur Heart J 1 (Suppl. B) pp 71-85
Serruys P W, Booman F, Troost G J, Reiber J H C, Gerbrands J J, Brand M vd,
Cherrier F and Hugenholtz P G 1982 IV. Symposium on Coronary Heart
Disease (Berlin: Springer) (in press)
Slump C H and Gerbrands J J 1981 Comp Graphics and Image Proc pp 18-36
Smith W M and Starmer C F 1976 Comp and Biom Res 9 pp 187-201
Starmer C F and Smith W M 1974 Proc. Comp in Card pp 143-7
Zir L M, Miller S W, Dinsmore R E, Gilbert J P and Harthorne J W 1976
Circ 53 pp 627-32

Some Imaging Requirements for Quantification of Structure and Function of the Heart

E L Ritman, J H Kinsey, L D Harris and R A Robb

Biodynamics Research Unit, Mayo Medical School, Rochester, Minnesota 55905, U S A

1. Introduction

The main purpose of this paper is to draw together some of our experiences in quantitative imaging of cardiac structure and function. The overall outcome of our experiences is that the spatial and temporal resolutions of the scanning procedure are more demanding (technologically) than are the spatial and temporal resolutions of the image that is generated from the scan data.

The scan data for this study were generated with the Dynamic Spatial Reconstructor (DSR), a multiple X-ray source, stop action, volume scanning imaging device (Ritman et al 1978, and Kinsey et al 1980) which utilizes the principle of computerized transaxial tomography. The patient or animal scanned is positioned inside the machine at the center of rotation as indicated in Figure 1.

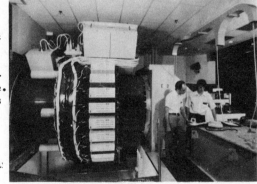
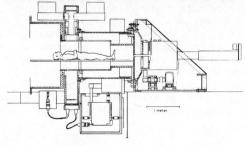

Figure 1 - Upper panel: Dynamic Spatial Reconstructor scanner assembly. The entire structure to the left of the men is cantilevered from the triangular base. Multiple image isocon TV cameras and corresponding X-ray sources are arranged along a vertical plane. Rotation of the cantilevered section increases the number of angles of view per scan in proportion to the programmed duration of the scan. Lower panel: Midline longitudinal section of the scanner shows relationship of human subject lying on table and the surrounding gantry (Reproduced with permission from Behrenbeck et al, Proceedings of the NATO Advanced Study Institute on Diagnostic Imaging in Medicine, In Press).

06/81/ELR

Fourteen X-ray tubes and 14 television cameras are attached to the scanner. The X-ray tubes are arranged 12° apart along a semicircular array with one television camera positioned directly opposite each X-ray source. As each X-ray tube is pulsed for 350 microseconds, a 30 cm x 30 cm image is generated on a fluorescent screen interposed between the subject and television camera. The corresponding television camera photocathode is gated on for 762 microseconds and the fluoroscopic image is recorded on the image isocon target for subsequent readout and recording on video disc. The data flow of the DSR system is illustrated in Figure 2. The 14 television images are

NON-INVASIVE NUMERICAL DISSECTION
(DSR Based Synchronous, Stop-Action Volume Scanning)

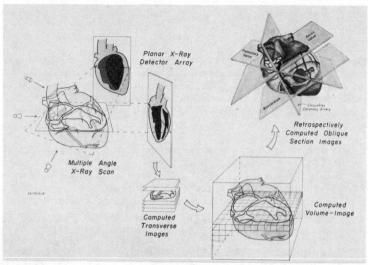

Figure 2 - Schematic flow chart of the sequence of procedures performed by the Dynamic Spatial Reconstructor system for generation of volume images which can be viewed following mathematical sectioning in arbitrary orientations and locations. X-ray images of the chest and its anatomic contents (e.g. heart) are recorded from many angles of view around the patient or experimental animal. This information is used to generate the data ("stack" of images of parallel transverse sections) required for a volume image using a reconstruction algorithm. Synthesis from up to 240 parallel, 1 mm thick, cross sections of the chest and its contents results in three-dimensional array of little cubic picture elements (voxels) each with a grey scale value. The final panel illustrates the need for sectioning this volume image in arbitrary orientations and locations. Parallel contiguous sections would be required for measurement of regional myocardial wall thickness. An oblique section would be required for measurement of pulmonary valve area, many multi-oriented adjacent (and often intersecting) contiguous sections may be required for visualization of coronary artery cross sections along the length of tortuous multioriented major branches of the coronary arterial tree. (Reproduced with permission from Ritman et al: Non-invasive visualization and quantitation of cardiovascular structure and function. The Physiologist 22(6):39-43 (December) 1979).

generated over an 11 millisecond period and are recorded in multiplexed
form on seven video disc channels at a repetition rate of 60 scans/second.
Each of   up to 120 horizontal scan lines of each of the 14 television
images is then used to reconstruct images of the corresponding 120 transverse cross sections. The video signal is digitized with a real-time
analog-to-digital converter and the -ray intensity data normalized for
the nonuniform distribution of the overall detection system. In this
manner, a "stack" of 120 cross section images is generated for each 1/60
second of the duration of a scanning sequence (up to 20 seconds).

There are four major aspects to the DSR design. First, the device scans a
volume so as to permit measurement of, for instance, muscle mass and chamber volumes. These values are obtained from a three-dimensional array of
picture elements (voxels) referred to as a volume image of a cylindrical
volume approximately 21 cm in transverse diameter and 21 cm in cephalocaudal height. Second, the volume is scanned by means of multiple
parallel transverse sections but accurate and meaningful measurement
(in a pathophysiological sense) can often only be obtained from images of
oblique sections through the body (see Figure 3). Such oblique sections,
with the correct orientation (e.g. normal to the vessel lumen) and location (e.g. through a valve orifice) in the organ or structure of interest, are computed retrospectively from the volume image (Harris 1981).
The spatial and density resolution of the volume image is comparable in
all three orthogonal directions. Third, the volume is imaged within a
sufficiently brief period of time such that the motion of the structure of
interest is less than about one resolution element. The DSR is designed
to have maximal spatial resolution of approximately 1 mm in the heart.
This speed is based on the observation that the endocardial surface moves
at up to 100 mm/sec in the transverse plane during peak of the systolic
ejection phase. Fourth, the images are generated at sufficient repetition rate for a sufficient period of time so that cardiogenic motion can
be quantitated. The retrospectively programmable analysis of DSR data
has enabled the exploration of the independent roles of spatial and temporal resolution of the scanning procedure and of the images.

Figure 3 - Schematic diagram of
volume image (stack of parallel
thin slices) generated by DSR.
Quantitative analysis of coronary
diameter, aortic diameter, wall
thickness, etc., all require
computation of images of oblique
section which goes through the
structure of interest at the
required angle and location.
(Reproduced with permission from
Sinak et al: Dynamic Spatial
Reconstructor. In Higgins,
C B: Computerized Transmission
Tomography of the Heart and
Great Vessels - Experimental
Evaluation and Clinical
Application (In Press)).

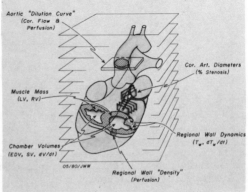

MULTI-FACETED EVALUATION OF
MYOCARDIAL ISCHEMIA
Measurements Made from DSR Image Data
(Volume Image, 0.01sec, 60/sec)

2. <u>Role of Spatial and Temporal Resolution of Scanning Procedure Versus</u>
   <u>Role of Spatial and Temporal Resolution of Images Derived from Scan</u>
   <u>Data</u>

The implications of these four requirements can be readily expressed in
terms of spatial, density and temporal resolution needs if, for instance,
DSR-based measurements correct to within 10% are desired. However, a less
tangible requirement is granularity needs, that is, how accurately does a
time "window", pixel location or slice location have to be controlled. As
will be shown later, the spatial and temporal granularity needs of the
<u>scanning</u> procedure are far more stringent than the spatial and temporal
resolution of the data conveyed by the images. The following discussion
examines the role of slice thickness and scan aperture time on accuracy of
measurements of the heart.

2.1 <u>Spatial Resolution</u> - A 10 mm thick slice may introduce a major problem due to the partial volume and sparse sampling effects. These disadvantages have to be weighed against the gain in signal-to-noise of the
image.

(a) <u>Photon Capture</u> - The thicker the slice the greater the number of
X-ray photons "captured" per picture element (voxel). This effect is
demonstrated in Figure 4. Minimum slice thickness is established by X-ray
detector thickness. Total slice thickness of image is determined by addition of contiguous scanned slices.

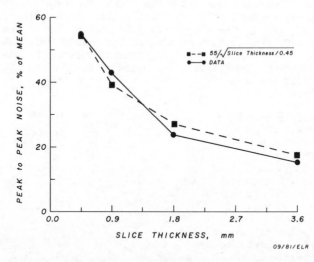

(9 cm Plexiglas Phantom, 90 KV, 6 mA-s, 104 Views)

<u>Figure 4</u> - Variability of estimated myocardial roentgen opacity was evalu-
ated in a 15 kg dog. Slice thickness of imaged transverse (and retrospectively computed oblique) section was increased as indicated along abscissa.
Sampled area of 0.25 cm^2 contained 100 pixels. The dashed line is
analytically computed square root function of slice thickness. These data
quantitatively confirm the visual improvement in image quality associated
with increased slice thickness.

(b) <u>Partial Volume Effect</u> - If a scanned slice happens to pass partially pass through an anatomic structure of interest, the partial contribution of the structure and its surroundings would result in impairment of the effective density and spatial resolution of the structure. This effect is illustrated in Figure 5.

(c) <u>Sparse Axial Sampling</u> - A major concern is lack of axial resolution due to limited number of slices in the axial direction. As a consequence, spatial resolution is greatly impaired   at right angles to the scan plane. Often a long axis view (or 4 chamber view in sector echo terminology) is desired. If 1 cm thick transverse slices are scanned, an axial resolution of 1-1.5 cm would result and this would rarely be adequate for anything but gross approximation of cardiac anatomy. Estimates of regional anatomy (e.g. radius of wall curvature in sagittal plane)

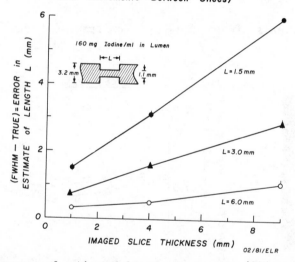

ROLE OF CT IMAGE SLICE THICKNESS IN ESTIMATE OF LENGTH OF STENOSIS IN CORONARY ARTERY
(88% Stenosis in 3.2 mm Diameter Lumen — 1 mm Increments Between Slices)

<u>Figure 5</u> - Accuracy of estimated length of stenosis (88% narrowing of 3.2 mm diameter lumen) as indicated by error of estimate which increases with imaged slice thickness. Slice separation remains 1 mm, i.e. for slices thicker than 1 mm there is overlap of slices; hence, the role of sampling interval plays the same role for all slice thicknesses. In all instances, the higher the concentration of roentgen contrast agent, the greater the accuracy. These data quantitatively indicate the detrimental role of increased slice thickness due to the partial volume effect. This effect tends to negate the increased resolution that accompanies increase in slice thickness (see Figure 4); hence, each structure under consideration must have a certain thickness at which these two opposing effects of partial volume blurring and increased photons per voxel cancel out optimally. (Modified with permission from Behrenbeck et al, Proceedings of the NATO Advanced Study Institute on Diagnostic Imaging in Medicine, In Press).

would probably be very poor, although reasonably accurate estimates of
global anatomy such as left ventricular muscle mass may be possible. This
is illustrated in Figure 6 which shows that if the volume (mass) of myocardium is to be estimated, as few as 8-10 strategically placed tomographic images will be adequate. However, great care must be taken that the
slices are at right angles to the long axis of the left ventricle. The
problem of near coplanarity of scan plane and heart wall can be partially
overcome by positioning the patient so that the long axis of the heart is
roughly at right angles to the scan plane. This does not help much at the
apex of the left ventricle but could help for the basal one to two thirds
of the ventricle.

(d) <u>Granularity</u> - If the slice is oriented and positioned appropriately
(i.e. with adequate "granularity" (or precision) of slice positioning),
the images can serve their purpose well. In other words, it may be important to position a slice accurately to within 1 mm even if a 1 cm thick
slice is acceptable with respect to partial volume effects once positioned
correctly. For instance, if a slice is oriented in the plane of the
mitral valve just on the apical side of the mitral valve ring, it could be

(Measurements from X-Ray Images of Heart Slices)

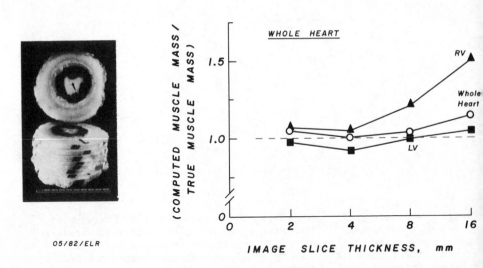

05/82/ELR

Figure 6 - A dog's heart was filled with dilute contrast agent in gelatin
and stabilized in a urethane foam. After the gel set, the heart was
sliced into 2 mm thick slices and an x-ray plate made of each one. These
pictures were used as "perfect" CT images of the heart. Slice thickness
could be increased by super-imposing the required number of slices before
making x-ray picture. The x-ray pictures were analyzed with a planimeter
to calculate wall mass and chamber volume by Simpson's rule. Increase of
slice thickness beyond a certain thickness (the thickness depends on the
size and detailed shape of the cardiac chamber) resulted in an increased
error of the estimate. These data quantitatively indicate the role of
sparse sampling on accuracy of volume estimates.

useful for evaluating myocardial perfusion or wall thickening even if 1 cm
thick. However, if the slice extends only 1 mm into the atrium, then the
density resolution is greatly impaired and the imaged grey scale within
the myocardium would be of questionable value for evaluating myocardial
perfusion.   This is due to the partial, but unknown, contributions of
muscle and atrial blood.

In addition to the roles of slice thickness and number, the size of the
volume scanned is important. Most adult left ventricles are around 10 cm
long - many are longer, hence the need to position accurately the
cephalocaudal extent of the volume scanned relative to the ventricle
increases the smaller the volume scanned. With small volumes (indeed, a
slice is the smallest volume), this will almost certainly have to be a
trial and error procedure, generally combined with trying to orient the
patient's ventricular long axis as close to right angles to the scan plane
as possible. This iterative positioning procedure could result in
increased exposure to radiation. This also presents a problem when progress of a pathological process (e.g. infarct size) is to be quantitated
with sequential scans. With the sparse sampling and poor granularity
(precision) of a slice positioning and angular orientation, it could be
quite difficult to be sure that the same "cut" is being imaged. Hence,
sequential comparisons of infarct size might be impossible in an adequately quantitative manner.

2.2 Temporal Resolution - A 100 msec scan duration may be quite adequate
for providing the necessary X-ray phase for adequate spatial and density
resolution. However, loss of resolution due to motion blurring has to be
weighed against increase in resolution characteristics which depend on the
duration of the scan for adequate photon capture.

(a) Scan Aperture Duration - A 50 msec scan aperture would generally be
an adequately short time to minimize blurring at most phases of the cardiac cycle (see Figure 7) if the slice plane is oriented at right angles
to the long axis of the left ventricle. If the scan plane and the left
ventricular wall plane (e.g. posterior wall) are nearly coplanar, motion
of the wall along the scan plane can be several times its radial velocity
(e.g. 60 mm/sec) because velocity in the scan plane = $(1/\sin(\theta))$ x
(60 cm/sec), where θ is the angle between the scan plane and plane of wall.
Hence, correct angle of the scanned slice, relative to the long axis of
the ventricle, is crucial if temporal resolution is to be used to maximum
advantage. This instance illustrates the critical interdependence of the
spatial, density, and temporal resolution and granularity. However, even
if it has the optimal geometric arrangement, the permissible aperture time
depends to a large extent on the timing of the aperture relative to the
biological motion that occurs during the scan aperture.

(b) Temporal (or phase) Granularity - A 50 msec scan aperture at end-diastole is satisfactory if the end of the scan is completed prior to onset
of systole. If the scan duration (aperture) extends partially into the
sustolic phase there is blurring. It is unlikely that the 50 msec
intervals will always fall at the appropriate times during the cardiac
cycle. Granularity (or temporal precision) of less than 10-15 msec is
requried to minimize this problem. Finally, the fact that adjacent slices
are scanned sequentially means that completion of the scan of the basal
slice would occur 200 msec after the onset of the apical scan. As an
 tire systole or rapid filling phase can occur in 200 msec, the imaged

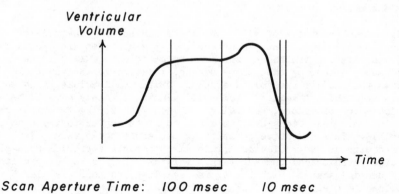

SCAN   APERTURE   TIME   DURING   WHICH
Imm   MOVEMENT   OF   MYOCARDIUM   OCCURS

Ventricular
Volume

Time

Scan Aperture Time: 100 msec   10 msec

Figure 7 - Schematic diagram of left ventricular volume during a cardiac
cycle. A long scan aperture time can be tolerated during diastolic but
only a brief aperture time can be tolerated during systolic ejection.
Nonetheless, even though a long scan aperture time can be tolerated in
diastole (i.e. minimal motion blurring), it is important that this long
scan aperture be positioned (in time) within a much smaller time interval
(e.g. 10 msec) than the length of the scan aperture.

three-dimensional shape of the left ventricle could be quite wrong - that
is, it never exists at any one time.

2.3 Density Resolution - In cardiovascular imaging using roentgen CT,
contrast agent will generally be used to delineate blood/tissue interfaces
and to indicate movement of heart. As shown in Figure 8, concentrations
of contrast medium causing 100% increase in roentgen attenuation are quite
readily achieved with 0.5 - 1 ml/kg contrast agent injected intravenously.
This translates to a need for approximately 5% density resolution based on
the assumption that 15% (some say as much as 30%) of myocardium is blood.
Hence, a 100% increase in blood opacity becomes a 15% increase in myocardial opacity. A 5% density resolution could therefore allow at least three
levels of contrast agent dilution to be distinguished. With this rather
modest imaging requirement, the spatial and temporal resolution requirements can be enhanced at the expense of density resolution.

3. Conclusion

When all these factors are considered, the objective characterization of
a cardiac scanner is difficult. An attempt has been made to cope with
this problem and the results, for the DSR, are shown in Figure 9. The
role of spatial granularity is conveyed in detail; however, the role of
temporal granularity cannot be well conveyed in this graph. For an object
that is moving at a certain rate, the upper (solid) lines would be curved
with a maximum located along the abscissa at a location dependent on the
speed of the motion. Experience with the DSR indicates (Behrenbeck et al

Journal of Computer Assisted Tomography, In Press) that, for objects
moving at 80 mm/sec, the resolution is maximum at the third data point
from the left along the solid line. Resolution for point 4 is less than
that indicated in this Figure.

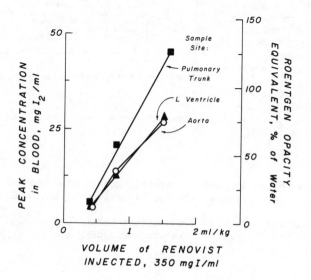

Figure 8 – Bolus of contrast agent injected into the femoral vein of a dog
was sampled in the pulmonary artery, left ventricle, and aorta and concentration of contrast agent in blood measured. Injection in the right atrium
instead of the femoral vein would result in higher concentrations of contrast agent in the aorta (Data courtesy of Dr R Padiyar).

Figure 9 - High contrast spatial resolution of the DSR as it is affected by increased voxel size and/ or number of angles of view (larger scan duration). The 0.15, 0.5 and 0.75 mm pixel size refer to the pixel size at the time of reconstruction. Moreover, a voxel size could be achieved by increasing slice thickness or by adding pixels (along the planes of the resolution elements). These data show that a reconstruction pixel size of less than 0.25 mm would probably result in increased resolution. These data also show that increased independence of new data (add. angles > add. slices > add. pixels) results in increased resolution. The abscissa is an index of radiation flux per voxel.

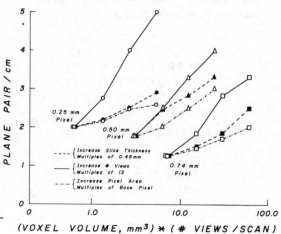

(DSR, 9 cm Plexiglas Phantom, 90 KV, 6 mA-s, Air Contrast)

(VOXEL VOLUME, mm³) ✳ (# VIEWS/SCAN)

Acknowledments

This work was supported in part by research grants HL-04664 and RR-00007 from the National Institutes of Health, Bethesda, Maryland 20014.

The authors would like to thank Mrs Darlene Kasten and Ms Julie Lauer and their colleagues for their assistance in typing and illustrations, respectively.

References

Behrenbeck, T, J H Kinsey, L D Harris, R A Robb, and E L Ritman: Three-dimensional spatial, density, and temporal resolution of the Dynamic Spatial Reconstructor. Journal of Computer Assisted Tomography (In Press)

Behrenbeck, T, L J Sinak, R A Robb, J H Kinsey, and E L Ritman: Some image characteristics of the Dynamic Spatial Reconstructor X-ray scanner system. Proceedings of the NATO Advanced Study Institute on Diagnostic Imaging in Medicine meeting. Castelvecchio Pascoli, Italy, October 11-24, 1981 (In Press).

Harris L D: Identification of the optimal orientation of oblique sections through multiple parallel CT images. Journal of Computer Assisted Tomography 5(6):881-887 (December) 1981.

Kinsey, J H, R A Robb, E L Ritman, and E H Wood: The DSR - a high temporal resolution volumetric roentgenographic CT scanner. Herz 5(3): 177-188 (June) 1980.

Ritman, E L, R A Robb, S A Johnson, P A Chevalier, B K Gilbert, J F Greenleaf, R E Sturm, and E H Wood: Quantitative imaging of the structure and function of the heart, lungs, and circulation. Mayo Clinic Proceedings 53:3-11, 1978.

Digital Radiography in Cardiac Imaging

S J Riederer
General Electric Co., Medical Systems, Milwaukee, WI USA

Abstract. Digital radiography systems are reviewed. Configurations
can be categorized according to detector geometry—area or linear.
Such systems are typically used with either energy or temporal subtraction techniques. Because of relative ease of implementation,
available x-ray intensities, and potential for 30 Hz imaging, temporal
subtraction in association with area detectors has thus far been the
method of choice for cardiac applications. Several technical aspects
of cardiac digital fluorography are discussed including imaging rate,
available intensities, and processing techniques. Clinical applications are discussed.

1. Introduction

A variety of systems have been developed recently which use x-rays as the
radiation source and ultimately express the final image in a digital
format. The range of applications pursued thus far has principally been
focused on the cardiovascular system but both nonvascular contrast and
noncontrast procedures have also been studied. More recently digital
radiographic systems have been applied to cardiac imaging. The procedures
studied have included ventriculography, assessment of coronary artery bypass grafts, assessment of congenital defects, and visualization of the
native coronary arteries. All of these procedures can be done with
intra-arterial contrast administration. Presently, however, there is
considerable research interest in achieving comparable or slightly
inferior but still diagnostic performance with intravenous contrast
administration. In this paper we review some fundamental concepts of
digital radiographic systems and subtraction techniques, discuss some
technical aspects of digital fluorography used with temporal subtraction,
and finally discuss some clinical results.

2. Review of Digital Radiography Techniques

Most digital radiographic techniques can be categorized according to
detector geometry and the type of subtraction performed. Geometries
used can be described as either linear or area. The subtraction methods
employed have included temporal, generalized temporal (temporally
filtered), dual-energy K-edge, dual-energy non K-edge, three-energy
K-edge, and hybrid subtraction. Recently Riederer (1982) has extensively
compared digital radiography systems applied to intravenous angiography.
Here we review some of the fundamental differences among geometry and
subtraction techniques.

2.1 Detector Geometry

The two principal generic geometries of digital radiographic systems are
area and linear. Flying-spot or point scanners have also been proposed
by Bjorkholm (1981) but thus far their use has been limited and their
slow imaging speed precludes many cardiac imaging situations.

Linear detector systems had their origin in part from computerized
tomography. In CT the patient is positioned in the gantry and the tube
and detector are rotated around the patient. For radiographic, rather
than CT, applications the patient is translated on the table through the
gantry whilst the tube and detector remain fixed. Successive x-ray pulses
correspond to adjacent lines of the image and the final image is constructed by the juxtaposition of several hundred lines. In addition to
this modified CT scanner approach of Brody (1980) several specifically
radiographic (non-CT) systems are also being constructed and studied, such
as that of Sashin (1979).

The second major geometry classification is the area detector. Digital
Systems studies have included the digitization of film, and perhaps most
commonly, the use of an image intensifier coupled to a digital television
system.

A comparison between area and linear geometries can be made based on
several parameters important in x-ray imaging. First of all, because
of the added dimension the area detectors are far more efficient in their
use of available x-ray intensity emitted from the x-ray tube. This is
particularly important when x-ray statistical requirements are very
demanding, such as the visualization of small contrast amounts in small
arteries. On the other hand the wide area detection can be a limitation
because of the detection of high intensity x-ray scatter. For
example the scatter-to-primary ratio can be 3:1 or higher with area
systems while for linear detectors scattered radiation may comprise only
a few per cent of the total signal. In addition to tube efficiency and
scatter susceptibility a third important parameter is imaging rate. For
linear systems the scanning speed is typically no higher than 50-100
mm/sec, or equivalently, the time required per image is several seconds.
On the other hand the image intensifier television system can operate at
up to "realtime" video rates, 30 frames/sec.

2.2 Subtraction Methods

Most conventional methods in x-ray imaging do not employ subtraction.
Typically when the x-ray exposure is made the archival image, a film,
is simultaneously exposed and then subsequently developed. In digital
radiography on the other hand, images are stored in digital format during
acquisition and viewed prior to actual filming. Because the digital
storage is highly precise, and fast processing and transfer rates are
available, a variety of image manipulation routines are possible which
are considerably more cumbersome and time-consuming with film. These
routines include windowing (contrast enhancement), temporal integration
or averaging, temporal and spatial filtering, and subtraction. Subtraction in particular has   proved   to be useful in improving the
perceptibility of specific materials in a radiographic image.

Temporal subtraction is the most elementary and widely-used of the sub-traction methods. In this technique a "mask" image is made of some vasculature of interest prior to arrival of a contrast bolus. After the bolus arrives a second image is made and upon taking the difference the only non-zero signal is the distribution of the contrast agent. The sub-traction step is very sensitive and object contrasts of several percent or less can be successfully isolated. The major difficulty with temporal subtraction is susceptibility to motion. If a high contrast object, such as a bone, moves between the time the two images are made a motion artifact occurs for those points in which the bone is not registered. This undesirable residual signal can interfere with perception of the contrast bolus.

Energy subtraction is a technique which uses exposures made with two (or possibly three) different x-ray spectra. Because the attenuation coefficients of different materials, such as soft tissue and bone, behave differently from each other as a function of energy, appropriate subtraction can cancel the signals from some materials thereby enhancing those from others. A problem with dual-energy imaging of iodine is that the undesired contrast of soft tissue and bone cannot simultaneously be eliminated. Thus, unlike temporal subtraction, dual-energy imaging cannot provide complete isolation of iodine. Perhaps the major advan-tage of energy subtraction methods is that the exposures with the various spectra can be made within tens of milliseconds of each other, thus substantially reducing artifacts due to motion.

Finally, hybrid subtraction, proposed by Brody (1981), combines both temporal and dual-energy subtraction techniques. In this case low and high kVp exposures are made both before and during passage of the iodinated contrast bolus. A dual-energy image made prior to contrast can eliminate signals from soft tissue, yielding a bone-only image. Repeating the process for the contrast-filled exposures results in an image of bone and contrast. Finally, taking the difference between the two dual-energy difference images eliminates the bone contrast and provides complete iodine isolation. The advantage of hybrid over temporal subtraction is that the energy subtraction component can virtually eliminate the susceptibility to soft tissue motions such as those arising from peristalsis or swallowing.

2.3 Digital Subtraction Angiography

Both detector geometries as well as the variety of subtraction methods have certain advantages and disadvantages. To generate images of con-trast material at rates higher than, say, 1/sec, an area detector is preferred. In addition, if complete isolation of iodine is required, either a temporal or hybrid subtraction approach is desired. For the highest SNR per unit patient dose and for high frame-rate (30 Hz) capability, temporal subtraction becomes the method of choice. The association of a specific area detector, an image intensifier digital video chain, with temporal subtraction, is referred to as digital sub-traction angiography (DSA), at present the most commonly used digital radiographic method.

3. Some Technical Aspects of DSA

Thus far the principal applications of DSA have been in quasi-static situations, cases such as the carotid, renal, and peripheral arteries in which image rates of 1 or 2/sec are adequate. It should be recognized however that DSA systems have the capability to operate with continuous or rapidly pulsed x-ray exposures used in association with continuous video readout. Thus imaging at 30 interlaced video frames per second or 60 fields per second is possible. (It should be noted that not all commercial systems can operate at such high rates.) In this case the temporal subtraction sequence is initiated by first forming a mask image with a pre-contrast exposure. This image is digitized and stored in a digital frame memory. Several seconds later a continuous exposure commences and the video camera is read out at a 30 Hz rate. Synchronously with digitization of the video raster, the mask image is read line by line from the frame memory and the two images are digitally subtracted from each other. After subtraction the sequence of pixels comprising the difference image is digitally amplified, i.e. windowed, and then stored. At 30 Hz image rates the difference image is generally reconverted to analog format and stored on analog video disk. The result is a several second sequence of 30 Hz difference images. The data rate of the process is thus relatively high. For 512 x 512 images, compatible with 525-line video, at 30 images/sec the rate of the digitization and processing is in the realm of 10 MHz.

Spatial resolution of DSA systems is dictated by a variety of factors including matrix size, bandwidth of the video electronics, x-ray focal spot size, imaging geometry, and resolution of the image intensifier. At this time with 512 x 512 matrices, 5 MHz video bandwidth, and 1.0 mm focal spots the spatial resolution with respect to the input screen of the image intensifier ranges from 1.0 to 2.0 ℓp/mm for the 9 inch to 4.5 inch diameter field size of the image intensifier. Because of magnification the actual spatial resolution within an object is somewhat better.

Contrast resolution of DSA is principally determined by the number of detected x-rays, that is, DSA is principally quantum noise limited. For visualization of very small vessels, such as intracranial arteries, the detected air kerma must be in the realm of 9 Gy or about 3×10^7 detected x-rays per square cm. As the vessels of interest increase in size the statistical requirements can be relaxed. For example with ventriculography a typical procedure could operate at 0.17 μGy detected per frame at a 30 Hz frame rate. This is equivalent to about 2×10^8 detected events in a 20 cm x 20 cm field.

The DSA values themselves are potentially useful in quantitative applications. Kruger (1981) has shown that if the video waveform is amplified logarithmically the resultant signal is proportional to the projected amount of contrast material. Thus, to first order, if a DSA image of the left ventricle is integrated, the sum of the values is proportional to the ventricular volume. This can potentially be used in determining ejection fraction from a 30 Hz image sequence.

It was mentioned earlier that a limitation of area detectors is the acceptance of x-ray scatter. DSA is no exception despite the fact that a difference is being performed. Kruger (1981a) has shown how scatter modulates the iodine signal in DSA, an effect later experimentally verified by Riederer (1981). Nalcioglu (1981, 1982) more recently has shown how scatter if uncorrected can cause underestimates of ejection fraction and secondly,has proposed correction means. The magnitude of this effect is comparable to that in nuclear medicine ventriculography.

4. Digital Radiography Clinical Applications in Cardiology

Since the introduction of DSA by Kruger (1979a) and Ovitt (1979) and the earliest clinical work by Christenson (1980), Crummy (1980), and Meaney (1980), cardiological applications have been studied. However,more typically,DSA procedures have been limited to relatively static situations such as imaging the carotid, cerebral,renal and peripheral vessels as reported by the above investigators.

As discussed in Section 3, DSA systems can potentially operate in real time permitting image rates up to 30 Hz. Ventricular imaging at such rates was studied in detail with dogs by Kruger (1979b) using temporal subtraction derivative imaging and by Houk (1979) with rapid dual-energy subtraction. In both cases ventricular chamber dynamics were studied with intravenous (IV) contrast administration. Such techniques were next extended to humans and because of the digital nature of the data it was logical to study the accuracy of quantitative evaluation of ejection fraction. Nalcioglu (1981) and Shaw (1982) have studied the effects of x-ray scatter and the veiling glare of the image intensifier system and proposed means for correction. At this time high quality image sequences of the left ventricle can be obtained routinely with commercial systems and IV technique but quantitative work is still under evaluation. A second cardiac application is the assessment of congenital heart defects, studied by Buonocore (1982) using intravenous contrast injections. A potential limitation of this technique is the superposition of contrast-filled vessels and heart chambers on the area of interest.

Turning to smaller vessels, the assessment of patency of coronary artery bypass grafts is another potential application of DSA. Results to date, however, have not been consistently diagnostic with intravenous contrast injection as discussed by Guthaner (1982) and Ovitt (1982). In addition to the small vessel size and overlapped ventricles, another limitation is from the overlapped pulmonary vasculature. Such structures not only opacify but are approximately the same size as the grafts themselves. Any slight motion yields motion artifacts which can mimic the grafts.

Finally,even in the early work of Kruger (1979a), the native coronary arteries were imaged in dogs with IV studies, but thus far there has been little success with humans. Among the advanced methods being studied are low-pass spatial filtering by Mistretta (1982) and temporal filtering by Kruger (1981b).

To summarize IV studies, ventricular imaging is almost routine, although quantitative use of such images is still under study. Imaging of native coronary arteries and coronary artery bypass grafts is only occasionally successful.

When DSA is used with intraarterial (IA) contrast administration many of the problems associated with the IV procedures are suppressed or eliminated. In particular, the contrast levels are much higher and, because of the selectivity of injection site, often only the vessels or chambers of interest opacify thus alleviating the problems of superposition. Ventriculography with an IA approach is virtually routine and Brody (1981) has reported successful imaging of the coronary arteries with selective injections. Using short temporal integrations, Kruger (1982) is studying the use of decreased amounts of contrast material to visualize coronary arteries. Indeed, perhaps the largest obstacle to routine DSA IA imaging of coronary arteries is the vast data storage required; e.g. 20 sec at 30 Hz requires 600 frames of storage.

To summarize, DSA cardiac studies have markedly superior spatial resolution and statistical precision than nuclear medicine. With IV contrast administration, visualization of the cardiac chambers is readily attainable while the imaging of smaller vessels is complicated by low contrast levels, superposition of other opacified regions and motion artifacts. For the IA case, except for some possible loss in spatial resolution DSA competes favorably in image quality with conventional film techniques.

5. Acknowledgments

The author acknowledges the support of General Electric Company, the invitation of the Hospital Physicists' Association, and the clerical help of Mary Koch.

References

Bjorkholm P, Annis M, Frederick E et al 1981, Proc. SPIE 273 103.
Brody WR, Macovski A, Lehmann L et al 1980, Inv. Radiol. 15 220.
Brody WR 1981, Radiol. 141 828.
Buonocore E, MacIntyre W, Pavlicek W et al 1982, Proc. Dig. Video Tech. in Cardiovas. Rad., Kiel.
Christenson PC, Ovitt TW, Fisher HD et al 1980, Am. J. Roent.135 1145.
Crummy AB, Strother CM, Sackett JF et al 1980, Am. J. Roent. 135 1131.
Guthaner D 1982, private comm.
Houk TL, Kruger RA, Mistretta CA et al 1979, Inv. Radiol. 14 270.
Kruger RA, Mistretta CA, Houk TL et al 1979a, Radiol. 130 49.
Kruger RA, Mistretta CA, Houk TL et al 1979b, Inv. Radiol. 14 279.
Kruger RA, Mistretta CA, Riederer SJ 1981a, IEEE Trans. Nucl. Sci. NS-28(1) 205.
Kruger RA 1981b, Med. Phys. 8 466.
Kruger RA 1982, private comm.
Meaney TF, Weinstein MA, Buonocore E et al 1980, Am. J. Roent. 135 1153.
Mistretta CA 1982, private comm.
Nalcioglu O, Seibert JA, Roeck WW et al 1981, Proc. SPIE 314 294.
Nalcioglu O, Seibert JA, Tobis JM et al 1982, Proc. Dig. Video Tech. in Cardiovas. Rad., Kiel.
Ovitt TW, Capp MP, Christenson P et al 1979, Proc. SPIE 206 73.
Ovitt TW 1982, private comm.
Riederer SJ, Belanger BF, Keyes GS and Pelc NJ 1981, Proc. SPIE 314 132.
Riederer SJ 1982, IEEE Trans. Med. Img. 1.
Sashin D, Sternglass EJ, Spisak MJ et al 1979, Proc. SPIE 173 88.
Shaw CG, Ergun DL, Myerowitz PD et al 1982, Radiol. 142 209.

Potential Applications of NMR in Cardiology

R A Lerski,　　　J S Orr and　　　R E Steiner*

Departments of Medical Physics and Radiology*, Hammersmith Hospital, London

Abstract. Recently, Nuclear Magnetic Resonance (NMR) imaging has been
shown to be a method of great diagnostic promise, both for brain and
body scanning. The physical principles of the technique are described
in some detail and the nature of the imaging process outlined with
regard to proton density and relaxation time (T_1 and T_2) images. A
brief discussion of the factors that determine these parameters in soft
tissues is given.

Potential applications of NMR in cardiology fall into four main areas.
Firstly, the heart can be imaged either with or without ECG gating and
functional information may be available. Secondly, information concerning blood flow can be obtained since the NMR signal from a moving
medium will vary depending on the time after excitation that data is
collected. Indeed, it should be possible to selectively image only the
moving material and receive no signal from the static structures. The
third area of application is the characterisation of the myocardium
from measurements of NMR parameters which may be able to distinguish
normal from infarcted or necrosed tissue. Lastly, relaxation times can
be affected by paramagnetic impurities and, because molecular oxygen is
paramagnetic, information with respect of oxygenation can be obtained.
It therefore appears likely that NMR will be capable of making a significant impact in several areas of cardiology.

I. Introduction – NMR Theory

Nuclear Magnetic Resonance relies on the exploitation of the fact that
nuclei with an odd number of protons or neutrons possess a net spin and
hence a magnetic moment and can interact with an applied magnetic field.
In zero field these nuclear magnets are orientated randomly but when a
field is applied there is a tendency to produce some alignment in the
field direction since this is the state of lowest energy.

In the quantum mechanical description of NMR (considering Hydrogen nuclei,
i.e. single protons) two energy levels are possible when observation is
carried out along the static field direction. These energy levels (Figure
I) differ in energy by $\Delta E = \gamma \hbar H_0$ where γ is the gyromagnetic constant, $\hbar$
is Planck's constant divided by 2π and H_0 is the applied static magnetic
field. Transitions between these energy levels may be stimulated by elec-
tromagnetic radiation of frequency determined through the relation

$$\Delta E = \hbar \omega_0$$

hence　　$\omega_0 = \gamma H_0$, i.e. the frequency is directly proportional to the

applied field. For the nuclei of interest the frequencies lie in the radio-
frequency (RF) range.

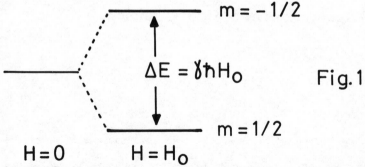

$$\Delta E = \gamma \hbar H_o$$

Fig.1

It is also useful to consider the normal populations of the energy levels
which at a temperature T are determined by the Boltzmann relation

$$\frac{n^-}{n^+} = \exp \frac{-\Delta E}{kT}$$

$$= \exp \frac{-\gamma \hbar H_o}{kT}$$

For an applied field of 0.1 Tesla (typical in NMR imaging) and temperature
of 300 K this ratio is very close to unity (in fact 0.999996), so that NMR
is a relatively insensitive technique. A consequence of this is that NMR
experiments may only easily be performed with abundant nuclei and signal
averaging must be employed to investigate less abundant species. At present and in the foreseeable future NMR imaging will continue to be
performed for Hydrogen nuclei (protons) whose abundance in the body is
unquestionable.

NMR experiments are usually described in terms of classical theory since
visualization of the experiment is rather simpler than in the quantum
theory. The classical description is valid because the energy difference
between the energy levels (ΔE) is much less than the Boltzmann energy kT
and because large numbers of nuclei (typically 10^{18}) are concerned. The
nuclear magnets are regarded as precessing at the Larmor frequency round
the static field direction (Figure 2),

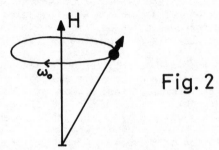

Fig. 2

this frequency being given by the same relation as above

$$\omega_o = \gamma H_o$$

The bulk magnetisation from a summation of all the nuclear magnets points along the static field direction. Now, the experimental situations that are to be described involve the bulk magnetisation being moved away from the static field direction (the Z axis) and this can be further simplified by observation in a rotating frame of reference whose Z axis is in the same direction as the static field but which rotates round this axis at the Larmor frequency (Figure 3).

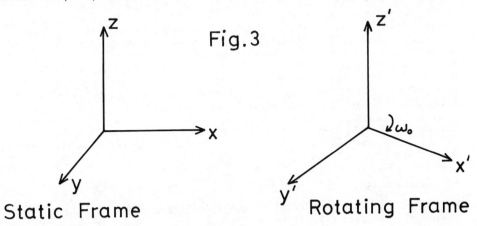

Fig.3

Static Frame   Rotating Frame

In this rotating frame the static field H_o disappears from the equations of motion and disturbances of the bulk magnetisation away from the Z direction are simplified since the precession around the Z axis has also been removed.

RF pulses applied in the XY plane can rotate the magnetisation to any direction, the angle of rotation for a particular pulse being determined by its duration (t_w) and magnitude (H_1), $\theta = \gamma H_1 t_w$
as shown in Figure 4.

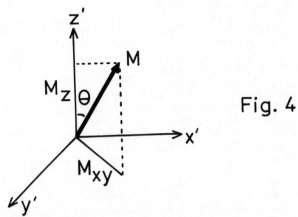

Fig. 4

After a particular RF pulse the system tends to relax back to its equilibrium configuration, the component M_z does this with a time constant T_1 (the longitudinal relaxation time) and the component M_{xy} with a time constant T_2 (the transverse relaxation time). These two parameters, together with the density of resonant nuclei, ρ, form the basic quantities measured in an NMR experiment.

Sequences (i.e. combinations of suitable RF pulses and data collection timings) may be designed to allow the measurement of any one of these
parameters with minimum influence from the others. A description of these
sequences is outside the scope of this article (see for example Gadian 1982)

Fortunately it turns out that the relaxation mechanisms that determine T_1
and T_2 in tissues are sufficiently different from each other that different
information is often contained in the two parameters. T_1 depends on an
energy exchange between the nuclear spins and the lattice (i.e. molecular
framework) whilst T_2 depends on exchange between the nuclear spins themselves. Generally, the relaxation mechanisms are stimulated by time varying
magnetic fields caused by, for example, molecular motion. As far as T_1 is
concerned this process is most efficient when the frequencies of these
molecular fields approach the Larmor frequency. The efficiency is also
high for T_2 at this frequency but, in addition, there is an important contribution from low frequency molecular motion.

Published clinical imaging studies have demonstrated these differences in
T_1 and T_2 images (Bailes et al 1982) but detailed explanations have not been
given.

2. NMR Imaging

NMR imaging systems measure ρ, T_1 and T_2 in whole bodies through an application of the basic principles outlined above. In addition, in order to
form the cross-sectional image, they use magnetic field gradients to give
positional information. Since the resonant frequency is directly proportional to the applied field it is possible to derive spatial information
from the frequency spectrum of NMR signals collected under the application
of linear field gradients. Several ways of applying these field gradients
are in use, suitable for scanning in different formats and reconstructing the
image using different algorithms. Typically such scanning gradients are
applied in the XY plane, with an additional larger gradient pulse being
used in the Z direction to selectively excite nuclei within the plane of
interest and move signals from either side of it outside the bandwidth of
the receiver. In the projection reconstruction approach a series of
gradients are applied in the X and Y directions to give 180 equally-spaced
projections through the object. These are then Fourier transformed and the
image reconstructed by filtered back projection in a manner analogous to a
translate-rotate X-ray CT system.

The principal components of an NMR scanning system are therefore a magnet
large enough to accept the human body, electronics to produce field
gradients, generate and receive RF pulse sequences and a computer to
collect the data and construct the images. The computer may be very
similar to the systems used for X-ray CT scanning since, as stated above,
the principles of image construction after data collection are essentially
the same.

The magnetic fields used for the static field range from about 0.04 Tesla
up to 0.35 Tesla with uniformities better than a few parts in 10^5 over the
imaging volume. This latter condition is required to minimise the dephas-
ing of the nuclear spins caused by field inhomogeneity and to keep the
system bandwidth low. The X and Y gradients used are very small, usually
only a few gauss over the imaging volume.

3. Applications in Cardiology

Possible applications of NMR in cardiology can be separated into four headings

(i) Cardiac imaging

Conventional NMR imaging sequences can produce cross-sectional cardiac images in any chosen plane. Figure 5 shows a proton density image across the right and left ventricles. Such images may either be ungated or gated to the cardiac cycle. A present disadvantage is that data collection times are rather long but it is

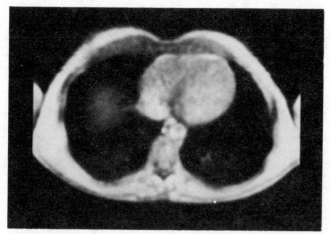

Fig.5

possible that functional information may be derived from these images.

(ii) Flow

In the previous section the slice selection technique was briefly described. Nuclei within the slice of interest experience a magnetic field of magnitude such that their resonant frequency is equal to the centre frequency of the RF receiver whereas nuclei outside the slice experience an additional field from the Z gradient so that their resonant frequency is shifted outside the receiver bandwidth. Figure 6 illustrates the situation.

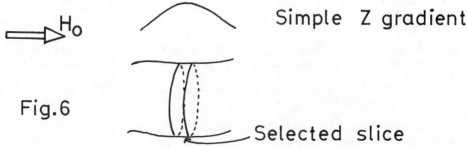

Fig.6

This description is only strictly valid in the absence of movement. Since data collection occurs in the NMR sequence after a delay from the slice selection, moving material could no longer be within the slice and the magnitude of the NMR signal from such moving material can vary depending on the exact time delay. Flow measurements using NMR have demonstrated sensitivity to 0.01 cm.sec^{-1} and rates up to 600 cm.sec^{-1} have been observed (Jones and Child 1978). Flow effects have been observed in work at the Hammersmith Hospital and it seems likely that measurements of cardiac blood flow will prove possible.

(iii) Myocardial characterisation

Measurements of T_1 and T_2 values have been shown to have a useful range in different tissues (e.g. Smith et al 1981) and it is to be expected that when methods for their accurate measurement from NMR images are developed they may be used as tissue characterising parameters. NMR cardiac images of the myocardium will be investigated to determine whether such measurements will be able to differentiate ischaemia from necrosis.

(iv) Oxygenation

NMR relaxation times are determined by molecular magnetic fields and hence magnetic impurities can have an important effect on their magnitude. In particular, paramagnetic impurities can be important since the unpaired electron magnetic moment is around 1000 times greater than the nuclear magnetic moment (see Dwek 1973). By a fortunate chance molecular oxygen is paramagnetic so that changes in the oxygenation levels of the blood can be seen in T_1 and T_2 values (Chiarotti et al 1955). Again it seems likely that this could have an application in cardiology where oxygen in the blood could be used as a 'constrast' agent for NMR. Difficulties may, however, arise in separating oxygenation effects from those due to flow.

4. Conclusion

Several possible applications of NMR imaging in cardiology have been identified, viz. imaging, flow measurement, myocardial characterisation and oxygenation studies. In all these areas work performed so far has been very preliminary but results have been encouraging and future work should lead to clinically useful techniques.

5. Acknowledgment

Financial support has been provided by the Department of Health and Social Security and the help of Gordon Higson and John Williams is gratefully acknowledged.

6. References

Bailes D R, Young I R. Thomas D J, Straughan K, Bydder G M and Steiner R E 1982. NMR Imaging of the Brain using Spin-Echo Sequences. Clinical Radiology 33 395.
Chiarotti G, Christiani G and Giuletto L 1955 Nuovo Clin 1 863
Dwek R A 1973 Nuclear Magnetic Resonance in Biochemistry (Oxford University Press).
Gadian D G 1982 Nuclear Magnetic Resonance and its Application to Living Systems (Oxford University Press).
Jones D W and Child T F 1978 NMR in Flowing Systems. Advances in Magnetic Resonance.
Smith, F W, Mallard J R, Reid A and Hutchison J M S 1981 Lancet May 2 963.

Physical Techniques in Cardiological Imaging: The Cardiologist's Conclusions

D J Rowlands
University Department of Cardiology, Manchester Royal Infirmary,
Manchester M13 9WL.

Ladies and Gentlemen, I am sure that few of us who have been present during this meeting will have failed to learn something of the physical principles used in cardiological imaging. Some of us however will not have had our views modified in certain areas. Those of us who are clinicians will, I believe, be more understanding of the capabilities and of the difficulties of imaging techniques from the physical viewpoint and hopefully the technologists will be more aware of the clinically relevant problems. In cardiology we need not only to be continually aware of developments which are occurring in all the available techniques but also to remain with our feet firmly on the ground when it comes to considering the possible useful applications. There is no point in developing techniques which the clinician manifestly does not require.

I have listed the major areas of clinical relevance to the adult cardiologist and to the paediatric cardiologist. In adult cardiology, coronary artery disease, hypertension, valve disease, arrhythmias and myocardial disease are the most important problems. For the paediatric cardiologist, congenital heart disease is obviously the most important. We have received no evidence to suggest that arrhythmias or hypertension are amenable to study by an imaging technique. As far as congenital heart disease is concerned, the most useful techniques over the years have been the plain chest X-ray, contrast angiography, ultrasound and nuclear techniques. It is quite clear that although the chest X-ray will still always be the first imaging investigation to be undertaken, two-dimensional ultrasound has overtaken all the other techniques and is without question the single most informative imaging procedure in this group of conditions. The need for contrast angiography has declined significantly and the contribution from nuclear techniques is relatively low. As far as valve disease is concerned, the most important investigative approaches involve first of all clinical judgement, secondly, the plain chest X-ray and, thirdly, ultrasound. These three approaches between them provide most of the information which is required. Contrast angiography is still needed in a proportion of cases. Nuclear investigative techniques provide little if any help. As far as myocardial disease is concerned, clinical judgement, the plain X-ray and ultrasound provide all the necessary information in the vast majority of cases. Dynamic studies of left ventricular function by nuclear angiography provide a useful supporting role.

Without question the number one problem remains coronary artery disease. We need to know in great detail about the anatomy of the coronary arteries, their pathology, the integrity of myocardial perfusion and the patterns of coronary arterial flow. Coronary angiography is likely to remain the definitive investigative technique in this field. Ultrasound plays at most a very small role in this area and infarct-avid scanning seems to be of very little help although the possibility that a resurgence of the use of fatty acids with modern radiolabels might make a contribution has to be considered.

Thallium scanning provides some useful information as a screening procedure but since neither the sensitivity nor the specificity of this technique seem likely ever to exceed 90%, its role in this area has to be fairly limited. It may be useful for patients where coronary angiography is contra-indicated or where the electrocardiogram gives less than useful information (as in the presence of bundle branch block). One of the most useful areas of application is in the assessment of myocardial perfusion in zones known to be supplied by a coronary artery which has a stenosis of uncertain significance. It is, in my judgment, of very limited value in clinical situations where a patient has chest pain of uncertain aetiology. If the thallium scan proves to be positive then the logical step is to proceed to coronary angiography to quantify and define the lesions. If the thallium scan proves to be negative the logical step is still to undertake coronary angiography since the sensitivity of the thallium scan technique is well below 100%.

As far as left ventricular function is concerned, radioisotopic techniques currently offer the best non-invasive approach to the problem. First-pass and equilibrium gated techniques are now well established and have been appreciably refined. There will always remain a major element of uncertainty about the absolute values given for left ventricular function in view of the inherent difficulty in deciding on the position of the edge in the left ventricular angiogram. Contrast angiography remains the definitive technique for assessing regional left ventricular performance but its major drawbacks are that it is highly invasive, it involves relatively high radiation dose and the technique itself is likely to influence the parameter which it sets out to measure.

To this extent the usefulness of these procedures is already mainly determined. A change in the extent to which they are used will depend upon refinements in technique and processing methods and this is perhaps particularly true with regard to nuclear techniques. Ultrasound techniques have evolved extremely rapidly in the last ten years and further developments are to be anticipated.

Perhaps the most exciting area of all involves the new techniques which are currently under development. Computerised X-ray tomography, digital radiography and nuclear magnetic resonance all offer enormous hope for the future. To my mind the most impressive images which we have seen at this meeting have been those provided by Dr. Ritman. To describe the results of these investigations as 'fantastic' and 'mind boggling' does not appear to me to be extravagant and the potential uses for these techniques, should they ever become generally available, are clearly vast.

The rate of development is such that one would anticipate the need for a further similar conference along these lines within the next few years.

Author Index